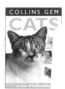

COLLINS GEM
CATS

a mine of information

COLLINS GEM
...hinese

COLLINS GEM
Classic
BOOKS

COLLINS GEM
Classic
FILMS

a mine of information

D1239496

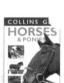

COLLINS G...
HORSES
& PONIES

COLLINS GEM
INSECT...

...KINGS
QUEENS

...LINS GEM
...SHROOMS
...TOADSTOOLS

a mine of information

COLLINS GEM
SNAKES

a mine of information

COLLINS GEM
SPIDERS

a mine of information

COLLINS GEM
STRESS
Survival Guide

a mine of information

COLLINS GEM
TAROT

a mine of information

COLLINS GEM
WINE
Guide

a mine of information

COLLINS GEM
WORLD
atlas

a mine of information

COLLINS GEM
YOGA

a mine of information

COLLINS GEM
ZODIAC
Types

a mine of information

COLLINS GEM

HOME
EMERGENCY GUIDE

The Printer's Devil

**Illustrations by
Roy Boyd**

HarperCollins*Publishers*

HarperCollins Publishers
PO Box, Glasgow G4 0NB

Created and produced by The Printer's Devil, Glasgow

First published 1998
This edition published 1999

Reprint 10 9 8 7 6 5 4 3 2 1 0

ISBN 0 00 472288 4

Printed in Italy by Amadeus S.p.A.

Contents

Appendices

> Note
> All measurements are given in
> metric. If you wish to use
> imperial measures, apply the
> following approximate
> conversions:
>
> 2.5 cm = 1 inch
> 1 metre = 3 feet
> 25 g = 1 oz
> 0.5 litre = 1 pint

Introduction

Ever wished you knew how to change a washer without calling a plumber; how to fix a blown fuse; or even just what to do to make your home a safer place? If you answered Yes, then this book is the solution to your problems.

The Collins Gem *Home Emergency Guide* is like an extra level of protection for your home. It tells you what you need to know instantly to put right something gone wrong, with remedial steps to treat the commonest home emergencies and advice on what you can do to make sure they don't happen again. Everything from your attitude through Fire and Infestations to basic First Aid is covered.

The Collins Gem *Home Emergency Guide* helps you limit damage and puts you back in control. It is an essential addition to any home library.

1 Coping

An Emergency: What Would You Do?

As we go about our daily business, most of us pass through different environments – work, school, shop, train or bus station, pubs and restaurants. We take it for granted that, if the need arose, someone in these places would take responsibility if something went wrong. From an event as trivial as a restaurant waiter spilling wine on your lap to a serious fire in a busy shop – plans are already in place to cope.

But could you take responsibility if the emergency were in your home? What would you do if a tap jammed on or your TV burst into flames? How would you limit the damage of coffee spilt on a woollen carpet? Domestic emergencies come in all sizes, from small and trivial to terrifying and potentially fatal.

Be prepared

You are the first line of defence against the many problems which inevitably crop up in the day-to-day running of your home. These problems may come on very suddenly, like a burst pipe or, like wet rot, take a much longer time to develop. Whether your problem presents in an instant or is longer-term, your response should be able to bring the situation within your control – minimising damage, curing the difficulty completely or, in a dangerous situation, allowing everyone in the house to escape with their life.

This book will provide you with the knowledge not only to deal promptly and confidently with many of the emergencies which may arise, but will give you preventative routines to follow and measures to take, where possible, to lessen the chances of dangerous or expensive emergencies ever confronting you in your home. You can start putting these routines into practice now.

Get informed

Everyone can always find more interesting things to do than read a book on how to protect themselves and their property. However, you should be aware that a better knowledge and understanding of how things work, the risks involved in their use and misuse and the possible dangers they present can even avert many emergencies before they arise.

The list on the next page lets you see in an instant which sections of this book are the very least ones you should read now. These will familiarise you with the most effective ways of coping with life-threatening situations. Your knowledge, or your ignorance, when confronting sudden difficulties in these areas literally could mean the difference between life and death. Don't wait for a problem to arise to find out how you would respond – train yourself now in how to cope.

ACTION!

SECTIONS TO READ NOW

Get insured

Thankfully, most of us will never have to
face a full-blown, bells-ringing emergency in
our homes. But householders will always

have smaller-scale domestic problems to cope with – from roof slates blown off in winter storms, to water damage caused by burst washing-machine pipes. Property problems are almost always unexpected, so it is wise to protect your building against them with suitable insurance policies.

As probably the biggest one-off purchase most of us will ever make, our houses should be treated to a level of financial and structural maintenance commensurate with their price-tags – yet many of us take more care to insure our cars than our homes. Insuring your home will help you financially to cope with any unforeseen problems which do arise and, more importantly, will allow you to create a safer, more comfortable environment for those who live there.

Do check carefully that any policy you choose covers all your needs – some do not cover infestation damage, for example, and you will need to seek out a dedicated policy from a reputable firm in that field.

Keep calm

Whatever the nature of the problem you face in your home emergency, your attitude to it will be all-important in determining whether you will cope successfully.

ACTION!

IN AN EMERGENCY

STOP – do not run about in a mind-fogging panic

THINK – five seconds' uncluttered thought will let you decide your main priority and how to achieve it, saving minutes of purposeless running about

ACT – when you have decided on a course of action, do it! Unless the situation around you is changing too rapidly, don't let yourself be sidetracked

2 Fire

ACTION!

EMERGENCY EVACUATION

1. If you can do it safely, close the door of the room where the fire is, and close other room doors as you move out

2. Feel with the back of your hand any closed door you need to open. If it's warm, don't open it – fire will be behind it. Never open any door to investigate

3. Gather everyone together and get them out immediately

4. If smoke is thickening, stay low – air is clearer near the floor

5. Once outside, stay out. Call the fire brigade on 999

Fire – How To Escape It

Fire is the most immediately life-threatening of home emergencies. Care and common sense are your most valuable weapons in dealing with it. This chapter shows you how to put them to good use in your home.

 FIRE FACTS

- There are around 60,000 house fires in Britain every year, killing more than 700 people and injuring over 9000

- Most deaths in fires come not from burning, but from toxic fumes and smoke, which poison or suffocate

- Modern building materials and house contents mean that a room can be totally ablaze in just 2 MINUTES

- Britain's top three fire causes are the careless use of chip pans, cigarettes and matches, and portable heaters

A Fire Escape Plan

The Emergency Evacuation procedure on page 15 is a simple set of instructions to help maximise your and your family's chances of escape in the event of a fire in your home. But it is no substitute for a properly thought-out Fire Escape Plan. Professional firms are legally obliged to have planned fire-escape routes and to practise drills, and there is no reason why you should not do the same.

Think ahead

Fire experts agree that the best time to plan your escape from a fire in your home is before it ever happens. Fires can move at devastating speed and it is hard to over-emphasise the debilitating effects of intense heat, noise, darkness, thick smoke, choking fumes, screaming children and your own indecision and rising panic. Action now could help you save your family from such a nightmare scenario in the future.

Plan ahead

You need to know how you would escape from each room in the house in turn, picturing in your mind how every member of your family could be got out in under two minutes. The Fire Escape Plan below shows the basics to consider; each of its aspects is dealt with in more detail in the following pages.

Fire Escape Plan

1. ESCAPE ROUTES: Decide on escape routes from every room by door and window, and how to use upper-storey windows

2. ESCAPE PROCEDURES: Tell everyone the safety rules for moving out through a burning building. Agree on an outside assembly point so an at-a-glance head-count can be done safely

Planning safe escape routes

Ideally, your best escape route is by a ground-floor door or window. But your scenario may well rule out that option, and your Fire Escape Plan should offer you alternatives.

Through rooms

 FIRE FACT
Most domestic fires start in the kitchen or living room

An educated guess will tell you that some rooms are safer to pass through than others. Does your plan allow for exiting through rooms other than the kitchen or living room?

Through doors

 FIRE FACT
Opening a room door to check on a fire inside can introduce enough oxygen to let the fire blow the door wide open

Doors can control the spread of fire through a house. Closing them behind you to separate you from the fire as you exit can give you the vital extra seconds you need to escape.

Conversely, doors left open will give fire a free run through your house. Worst of all is to open a closed door to a room where a fire is raging. The sudden entry of extra oxygen will not only stoke the fire up, but may well be enough to let it suddenly flare, throwing the door open and setting you ablaze.

There may be no sign that fire is raging within a room, so if you must check, or need to open a door to pass through, use this test.

Is it safe to open the door?

With the back of your hand, touch the door, or its metal handle. If either feels warm, leave it shut – fire will be inside.

NEVER use your fingers – the door could be hot enough to burn, and you may need to use your fingers to escape

Test with the back of your hand before opening a door

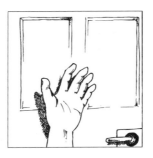

Through windows

Older-style double-glazing units which do not open can present unexpected obstacles if you are trying to escape a fire (see Danger! box, p.22). And if a window can be unlocked and opened enough to let you climb through, be sure always to keep its key nearby.

If you have to smash a window, cover the jagged bottom edge with a blanket or other thick item. One adult should go out and the

> ## DANGER!
>
> A double-glazed window unit cannot be broken like a normal window. If you cannot open your window enough to climb out, keep a heavy, sharp, pointed tool handy in the room to smash through the window at a corner

other stay in to pass children out in a safe, controlled way. If you are escaping through a high window, drop pillows and blankets onto the ground to break your fall. Hang to your full length from the window sill and then drop down. Hang children to their full length, gripping their wrists, before dropping them. **No-one should ever jump out of a window and never drop from above 1 storey**.

If you decide that your window is too high to escape from safely, you may decide to buy a fire-escape ladder (see pp.34–35).

Planning safe escape procedures

The rules for escaping a burning house are the same as those for the Emergency Evacuation

(see p.15). Having your Fire Escape Plan
thought out in advance will save vital seconds.

NEVER:

● *Investigate behind doors needlessly,*
  especially if you suspect fire is within

● *Stay behind to pick up belongings or*
  even pets – delays could cost you your
  life

Rehearse

Once you have decided on the various escape
routes, these escape procedures should form
the basis of your Fire Escape Plan. Discuss it
with your family and, as in business premises,
practise it regularly. Some of your planned
exits may be too risky to use except in an
emergency but if possible one person should
test them safely to make sure they are usable.

Make sure children know the Fire Escape
Plan, too – you could give them a floor plan

of the house, and ask them to draw how they
would get out of individual rooms if fire
began.

If fire breaks out in your home, you may
have only seconds to get everyone out.
Knowing your Fire Escape Plan will save
vital time and could be a life-saver.
Remember, planning and rehearsal are the
keys to your safe escape.

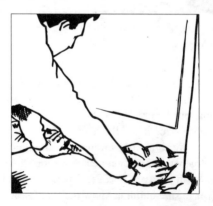

Sealing off a room when your escape route is blocked

If a safe escape route is blocked

Surviving in a burning house

1. Gather everyone together into a safe room, preferably with a phone to call the fire brigade

2. Close the door and wad it with towels or blankets. If there is a water supply in the room, soak them first

3. Open the window and shout for help until someone goes to phone the fire brigade. Smash a sealed unit (see pp. 21–22). Stay by the open window

4. If there is a water supply, douse the door and the walls nearest the fire while you wait for the brigade

5. On the first floor in a critical situation, assess your chances of dropping down (see pp.21–22). On higher floors, lean out for fresh air until the brigade arrives

Fire – How To Combat It
. . . .

Various equipment is available to help you
survive a fire in your home: to alert you, to
help you fight it and to help you escape.

To alert you

Your choice of fire-combatting equipment
will depend on your priorities, circumstances
and confidence, but first in line should be the
thing the fire brigade recommends as a
potential life-saver – a smoke alarm.

Smoke alarm

Smoke alarms or detectors are small, saucer-
sized boxes which are fixed to the ceiling. By
sensing smoke they detect fire in its earliest
stages, and emit a shrill alarm loud enough to
be heard at a distance, allowing you precious
extra seconds to escape. In a situation where
you have two minutes or less to get everyone
out, these seconds could be invaluable.

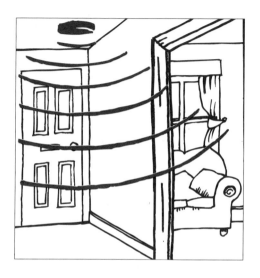

It is hard to overemphasise the speed at which a fire can spread and there is no guarantee that toxic fumes would not incapacitate you before you even suspected your house was on fire – a very real danger, particularly at night.

Unpopularity There is a considerable
resistance to the use of smoke alarms, largely
because of their perceived 'nuisance' factor –
regular maintenance is needed, and false
alarms are not uncommon – and because fires
are often seen as survivable. Although many
people are confident of their ability to detect
and escape fire, the 700+ British fire deaths a
year show that this is not always possible.

Maintenance In fact, the maintenance
involved in a smoke alarm is not great: a
monthly test and an annual battery change
will ensure it works properly. These few
minutes' upkeep are far less time than most of
us spend keeping our cars in working order.

False alarms Work in the house, including
DIY jobs and cooking, can set off a smoke
alarm. However, some models have an
override button which allows the alarm to be
disabled temporarily to allow you to do work
– for example, cooking a smoky meal –
which might otherwise set off the alarm.

Fitting Ideally, at least one smoke alarm should be fitted on each storey of your house. Fitting is simple and packs carry instructions. Any alarm you buy should carry a British Standards Kitemark. Do not fit alarms in the kitchen or bathroom, as steam and fumes set them off. 'Through' areas, such as the hall, at the foot of the stairs, and the landing at the top, are probably the best sites, as alarms there will be more easily heard. Individual alarms can be linked by an electrician, so a fire in one area will set off alarms elsewhere.

To help you fight

Before you try to tackle a fire, be aware of this safety rule: the safest course of action is always to evacuate the house immediately. When everyone is outside and you have rung the fire brigade, you will have to wait just minutes before the professionals arrive to fight the fire efficiently, confidently and with no danger to you or your family.

Fire extinguisher

If you are confronting a very small, containable fire and your family has already evacuated to safety, you may feel able to take on the fire yourself with an extinguisher. But before you do, consider the following comments, made by professional firefighters:

- professionals mistrust domestic extinguishers, which can foster a false confidence in the untrained

- you must know what type of fire you are facing before you use an extinguisher – you could imperil your life by using the wrong type for the job

- the amount of extinguisher in domestic units is enough to deal with only the very smallest fires

- the experts' advice is: if you cannot put the fire out in 30 seconds, get out of the building

FIRE FACTS: FIRE CLASSIFICATIONS

A Fires involving solid, usually organic material (paper, wood, fabric). The commonest type of fire

B Fires involving liquids or solids which liquefy (oil, petrol, paint, solid fat)

C Fires involving gases

D Fires involving metals

The table above shows types of fire. To use an extinguisher safely, you need to know which one works on each fire type. There are five:

- water (colour indicator: red)
- foam (colour indicator: yellow or cream)
- carbon dioxide (colour indicator: black)
- dry powder (colour indicator: blue)
- liquid gas & halon (colour indicator: green)

The table over shows which extinguisher is compatible with each fire type.

Fire Extinguisher Safety

	Water red	Foam cream	Co2 black	Powder blue	Halon green
A solids	✓	✓	✓	✓	✓
B liquids	✗	✓	✓	✓	✓
C gases	✗	✗	✓	✓	✓
D metals	✗	✗	✗	✗	✗
Electrical fires	✗	✗	✓	✓	✓

Use Your domestic extinguisher should be light enough to be liftable but heavy enough to have a useful capacity – consider around 1 kg and upwards. Always make sure that you position yourself between the fire and an escape route. Aim the nozzle at the base of the fire, and sweep the extinguisher from side to side across the fire as you use it. **Never tackle an electrical fire unless the power has been switched off at the mains.**

Maintenance Make sure your extinguisher is checked and serviced regularly according to the manufacturer's instructions.

Fitting Store your fire extinguisher in a place where you can get to it easily if fire breaks out. If you do have a fire, your extinguisher won't be much use in a cupboard.

Fire blanket

Fire blankets (about 1 m square) are meant to deal with small kitchen- or cooker-related fires, such as a burning chip pan or tea towel.

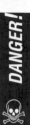

DANGER!

Old fire blankets made of asbestos, may be dangerous. Do not use it, or dispose of it yourself. Instead, check your blanket's safety with your local environmental health department, and get their advice on disposal.
See pp.254–255 for more details

Use Your fire blanket should simply be shaken out and dropped over the flames. Make sure it will cover enough to smother.
Fitting A wall mounting close to the cooker is best – but not behind it, so you don't need to stretch over the hob to get your blanket!

To help you escape

Fire-escape ladders

There are several fire-escape ladders on the market; check to see which one fits your needs. A well-thought out ladder, designed by

firefighters, is the flexible, shake-out metal
type which will lock into place when
unfurled. Ladders are available with a drop
of one (3.5 m) or two (6.5 m) storeys.
Use Escape ladders can be stored under your
bed until required. They can also be used in
conjunction with a separately bought child
harness which will strap a baby or small child
to a parent's body while allowing the parent
to keep both hands free for climbing down.

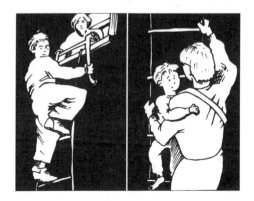

Fire – How To Prevent It

Despite the wide availability of fire-prevention equipment, the number of domestic fires in Britain is increasing all the time. Almost all of these fires are caused by the same conditions and domestic appliances.

 FIRE FACTS: THE TOP FIRE RAISERS

1. Chip pans and cookers
2. Portable heaters
3. Cigarettes
4. Matches and lighters
5. Faulty or mis-used electric wiring
6. Electric blankets
7. Blow torches
8. TVs and VDUs
9. Candles
10. Dirty chimneys

Chip pans

There are on average almost two chip-pan
fires an hour in Britain, from three main
causes – too much oil, overhot oil spilling
over onto the cooker, and wet chips. Avoid
chip-pan fires with this list of Don'ts and Dos.

> ✗ Don't ever leave the pan unattended
> ✗ Don't fill the pan more than a third full of oil
> ✗ Don't put the chips in if the oil is smoking
> ✔ Do dry the chips before putting them in

If your chip pan catches fire, this is what to do:

- turn off the heat
- drop a dampened tea towel, fire blanket
  or large pot lid on the flames (see p.38)
- NEVER lift the pan or throw water on it
- leave the pan to cool for an hour
- if you can't control the fire shut the door,
  get everyone out and call the fire brigade

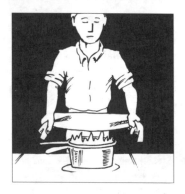

Cookers

Chip pans cause most cooker-related fires, but there are others, nearly all attributable to cookers accidentally turned on or left on.

✗ Don't leave pot handles jutting over other hot rings, or where children can grab them

✗ Don't let electrical flexes from other nearby appliances trail across the cooker surface

✗ Don't dry tea towels over the cooker

If your cooker or any electrical item catches fire, this is what to do:

- ◉ follow your normal escape procedure
- ◉ if your family is safely outside and if you can do so safely, turn off the electricity at the mains as you pass on the way out

Portable heaters

Heaters cause almost 3500 fires and around 60 deaths a year. The old, who use portable heaters relatively heavily, are more at risk.

> ✘ Don't put heaters near beds, sofas, curtains, cushions or other soft furnishings
> ✘ Don't use heaters to warm beds or clothes
> ✘ Don't sit closer than 1 m to a heater – if you doze your clothes or chair could catch fire
> ✔ Do keep heaters where they and their flexes won't be tripped over
> ✔ Do have an all-enclosing heater- or fire-guard if you have children

If your heater catches fire, follow the same procedure as outlined at the top of page 39.

Leaks from gas cylinder heaters can also cause fires, and even explosions. Be especially careful when changing cylinders – ensure good ventilation, in the open air if possible. Always turn portable gas and paraffin heaters off before filling or changing the cylinder or cartridge.

If fire breaks out near your portable gas cylinder heater, this is what to do:

- if you can, turn off the gas to the cylinder

- move the heater away if the fire has not yet reached it

- if the fire is too close, get far away from both the fire and the building containing it – the cylinder may explode like a bomb

- when you call the fire brigade, tell them that the fire involves a gas cylinder

Cigarettes, matches, lighters and candles

Cigarettes, matches, lighters and candles are responsible for starting more than 10,000 fires every year. This list of rules, once observed, should help keep you safe.

✗ Don't smoke in bed, or when you are tired

✗ Don't let a cigarette burn in an ashtray, even if you intend to come back to it – always put it out

✗ Don't leave any candle unattended

✔ Do empty and wash out ashtrays at night – this extinguishes smouldering embers and cuts down on smoky smells in your home

✔ Do store matches and lighters in a high cupboard where children can't reach them

✔ Do use candles in clear, uncluttered spaces away from soft furnishings

✔ Do keep lit candles away from ledges or other places children can reach

Electric wiring

Faulty wiring is one of the commonest home fire raisers and can surprise even those who are careful in most other respects. Experts say wiring should be changed every 25–30 years, but even if you don't have your whole house re-wired at its 25-year check, there are several modern safety measures you can have installed alongside existing circuitry which should cause minimum disruption. Probably the most important of these is a residual current device (see p.71).

There are several warning signs which should alert you to potentially flawed wiring:

- old, round-pin plugs and sockets
- bakelite socket covers
- hot plugs and sockets
- fuses blowing
- lights flickering
- brown burn-marks on plugs and sockets

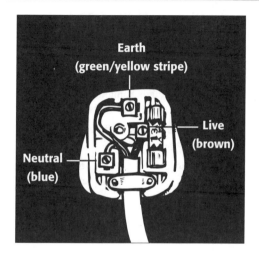

Wrongly wired plugs are another potential killer; the correct wiring is shown above. An easy way to remember wire positioning is by colour: bLue and bRown go Left and Right respectively, following their second letters; the striped wire, the earth, is left for the middle.

Remember also to use the correct fuse for

the equipment and try to avoid using adaptors
– the best rule is, one appliance, one socket.
Deal with electrical fires as follows:

- if possible, turn off the power at the
  mains (although at night you may need
  to leave it on to see your way out)
- evacuate the house following the Fire
  Escape Plan
- if the fire is containable, everyone else is
  safe and the power is off, smother the
  flames with a fire blanket or extinguisher
  (see pp.30–34)

Electric blankets

Electric blanket fires claim around 35 lives
each year, largely through faulty blankets.
Their Don'ts and Dos are shown opposite.

If your blanket goes on fire and you follow
the electrical fires procedure above, get out as
soon as possible afterwards as there may be a
risk of toxic fumes.

✘ Don't get into bed without first switching off your electric underblanket

✘ Don't mis-use electric blankets: never use an underblanket as an overblanket or vice versa

✔ Do tie your electric underblanket to the mattress

✔ Do get a blanket with an overheat-protection facility when you buy a new one

✔ Do have your blanket serviced annually

✔ Do store your blanket flat, and keep it dry

Blow torches and blow lamps

As with most appliances, these are safe if used carefully and kept in accordance with manufacturers' instructions. Used by DIY-ers, professionals and even cooks, blow torches should never be left on unattended and should always be switched off when not in use. Use them in a clear space, away from carpets and curtains, and always keep a suitable means of extinguishing handy.

TV and VDU fires

The total number of fires caused by domestic electrical appliances currently runs at around 4000 a year. Of these, fires in TVs and computer screens carry particular dangers of their own risks – explosion and toxic fumes.

Follow the general rules for dealing with electrical fires, but if you are in the same room as a burning TV or VDU, never stand in front of the screen – it could explode.

✗ Don't keep TVs or VDUs plugged in when they're not in use
✔ Do use screens in a clear, uncluttered area to allow maximum ventilation

Chimney fires

Unmaintained chimneys cause not just fires but also the more insidious danger of carbon monoxide poisoning (see p.56).

Chimney fires can be seen from the outside

usually before those in the house are aware of them, so do let the occupants know if you see sparks or flames coming from their chimney.

> ✘ Don't build up huge fires in the grate
> ✔ Do have chimneys cleaned yearly, preferably in autumn. Old birds' nests can be cleared before the fire is used intensively in winter

If your chimney goes on fire:

- call out the fire brigade
- clear carpets and furniture away from the hearth to avoid falling burning debris
- pour soapy dishwater into the grate – detergent will put out the fire quicker and steam will rise up to cool the fire in the chimney
- if the fire is not containable or the room is becoming too smoky, get out, closing doors and windows as you go

Clothing fire

One of the most terrifying fire accidents to confront is a clothing fire. You need to know what to do instantly to get the situation under control before disfiguring damage occurs. The principles to follow are the same, whether your clothes or someone else's, are on fire.

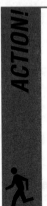

ACTION!

IF YOU ARE ON FIRE

1 STOP – moving fans the flames

2 CROSS your arms over your chest, with hands on shoulders to protect your face

3 DROP & ROLL slowly on the ground to put out the flames, or wrap yourself in a non-synthetic blanket, curtain or carpet

4 COOL the burns – sit in a cold-water bath. Don't pick off fabric stuck to your skin. Call 999

ACTION!

IF SOMEONE ELSE IS ON FIRE

1 STOP THEM

2 DROP THEM – by tripping if necessary

3 ROLL THEM – in a non-synthetic blanket, curtain or carpet

4 COOL THEM with water – sit them in a cold-water bath. Don't pick off fabric stuck to the skin. Call 999

Nightly fire patrol

To lessen the risk fatalities in your home as a result of fire, build into your pre-bedtime nightly routine a patrol around the house to check on possible places of combustion.

The suggested night patrol listed on the next page should cover most houses, but remember to add anything else which is particular to your own home.

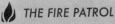 THE FIRE PATROL

- Extinguish cigarettes, empty and rinse out ashtrays, dampening recently extinguished butts
- Check that the cooker is off
- Turn off all fires; put fireguards up before an open fire
- Unplug all electrical appliances, especially computers and TVs
- Turn off lights, including outside ones
- Check that you know where everyone in the house is
- Close doors as you go
- Switch off your electric blanket before getting into bed

3 Gas

ACTION!

IF YOU SMELL GAS

1 NEVER switch on a light, or light a naked flame

2 Open windows and doors

3 Make sure no gas appliance has been left on unlit

4 If not, you probably have a leak. Turn off the main gas tap (see p.53), usually found in the meter housing

5 Call the gas company's emergency line, from a room well away from any gas smell

6 If you can't turn the tap off or a strong smell remains, evacuate the house and call the police

Natural Gas
••••••••••••••

Prepare for an emergency

For any large-scale gas-related emergency, you must make sure that you know in advance where your main gas tap is. For most houses, this will be in the box that contains the gas meter. (See the illustration opposite.) The gas supply pipe has a large handle with a spanner-like key on the end – this is the tap that switches the supply on and off. Turn it down as far as it will go – usually, when the gas is switched off the handle will end up parallel to the ground and at right angles to the upright gas pipe.

As with other domestic emergency control switches, it is worth while making the effort now to familiarise yourself with the mains gas tap's location – if you do have a full-scale gas emergency, you may have to be able both to find the tap and to operate it in the dark.

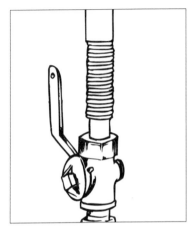

Gas main lever in the box containing your meter. To shut off the gas, pull the lever down through 90 degrees

Principles of gas safety

The two basic rules for dealing with any type of gas, as well as with its potentially dangerous by-products, are vigilance and care on your part and ensuring that there is always adequate ventilation around your heating appliances, and through the house in general.

Ventilation

Good ventilation is essential to ensure that any fuel-burning appliance works properly, so that any naturally ocurring harmful burn-off gases like carbon monoxide can be dispersed and drawn out of the room.

For this reason, rooms where any types of fire or a gas appliance are being used should never be sealed off completely from draughts. Chimneys, whether for gas, coal or wood fires, must be clean and well maintained, and any flue systems, which work by drawing in outside air and expelling harmful gas by-products, should be checked and cleaned regularly.

Vigilance

The lists of Don'ts and Dos in this chapter,
will help you to be a safe gas-user. In
practice, gas is one of the safest forms of fuel,
but this is achieved only by extreme care and
making safety an absolute priority. It also
pays always to be aware of the possibility that
something could go wrong at any time with
your gas supply – *never* take gas for granted.

Pointers to gas safety

- Gas is potentially deadly – never take chances with it
- Gas maintenance is not a job for the DIY-er – hire a registered professional
- Never use any appliance you have safety doubts about – have it checked
- Follow the list of Don'ts and Dos on p.57

Carbon Monoxide
••••••••••••••••••••

Gas leaks are frightening, but the gas supply has a built-in safety warning system – its noticeable smell. Far more difficult to detect, and far more dangerous, is a build-up of carbon monoxide. This colourless, tasteless and odourless gas is a killer of more than 50 people a year in Britain, with anything up to four times that number being hospitalised.

Causes

As a fire burns, it uses oxygen and emits carbon monoxide. This is normally discharged through a flue or a chimney, but if a fault develops the carbon monoxide can escape into a room. This may be because:

- a ventilation flue is blocked
- a room containing a gas appliance or fire has been sealed off from draughts
- an appliance is burning inefficiently

✗ Don't buy second-hand gas appliances not checked by a professional

✗ Don't run your car engine in a garage with the doors closed

✔ Do have your gas heating system and appliances serviced annually

✔ Do have adequate ventilation in any room or area where a fire is burning

✔ Do have all flues and chimneys cleaned annually and maintained properly

✔ Do buy carbon-monoxide detectors for each room, if you can afford them – but never rely fully on them

The list of Don'ts and Dos above should help minimise monoxide dangers in your home.

Sources

Of course, it is not just gas fires and appliances that burn carbon monoxide: any appliance which burns a fossil fuel can emit it, with coal gas actually being more dangerous than the usually mains-supplied 'natural' gas. Sources include:

- any open fire, including bonfires
- oil burners
- car-exhaust fumes

Signs

Students and those living in bed-and-breakfast or other rented accommodation who are dependent on someone else to ensure the safe maintenance of appliances, should be particularly alert to the warning signs below.

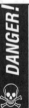

DANGER!

- Gas flames on appliances burning yellow or orange instead of blue
- Sooty stains on or above appliances
- A room that feels stuffy and airless
- Solid fuel appliances that burn slowly, or go out altogether

Symptoms

Never underestimate how toxic carbon monoxide can be. Its effects are so potent that even rescuers trying to save poisoning victims from affected rooms have been known to be overcome. Its symptoms include:

- drowsiness
- headaches
- sickness and diarrhoea
- stomach pains
- chest pains
- tiredness or weakness
- light-headedness, especially on standing

If these symptoms are noticed particularly in a specific room or part of the house, carbon monoxide poisoning must be suspected. In this case, switch off any fire or appliance and consult a doctor at once, even after you feel you have recovered.

The information below describes how to get monoxide victims out of a fume-filled room. Do not risk your own health in a rescue bid.

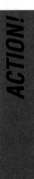

ACTION!

CARBON MONOXIDE AND TOXIC FUMES RESCUE

1 Open windows and doors

2 Drag the victim(s) outside, beginning with those most unconscious. Be alert to your own state throughout – cover your nose and mouth if needed

3 Loosen off restrictive clothing

4 Check for pulse or heartbeat. If none, begin emergency cardiopulmonary resuscitation (see p.233–6)

5 Leave the victim(s) in the recovery position (see pp. 236–7) and call an ambulance

Other Gases

The other gases most widely used in homes are types of LPG (Liquefied Petroleum Gas): butane and propane.

Butane gas is the type commonly used in metal cylinders to fire portable heaters. It is also used in lighters, some cordless hair tongs and for camping gas. Propane's storage requirements make it less suitable for domestic use, and it is not often used in British homes. Blowtorches can be fired by either type of LPG.

Both types of gas are odourless, but have an unpleasant gas-smell added to make leaks more easily detectable. Both are also toxic.

Be particularly careful when changing the cylinder on a portable heater. If you are unsure of the procedure, there is no shame in calling in a professional to show you how. *Never* take chances with any type of gas.

A list of Don'ts and Dos on the next page shows how to treat gas heaters with respect.

- ✘ Don't leave a heater or its cylinder where it can be knocked over – the cylinder's massive internal pressure could trigger an explosion in a faulty appliance
- ✘ Don't place a heater close to a bed, curtains or other furnishings
- ✘ Don't leave clothes in front of or draped over a heater
- ✘ Don't place a heater or cylinder in a corridor where it could block a fire exit
- ✘ Don't use portable heaters in a bathroom or a small room with poor ventilation
- ✘ Don't store cylinders in the basement – gas's heavier weight than air means leaks could remain undetected if underground
- ✘ Don't inhale LPG – it can asphyxiate
- ✘ Don't touch LPG – it burns like frostbite
- ✔ Do turn a heater off before you get into bed at night
- ✔ Do get your portable heater professionally serviced annually

4 Electricity

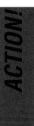

ELECTROCUTION

1 Switch off the current at socket or mains, whichever is quicker

2 Muscle spasms may make the victim grip the current source. Stand on a newspaper or in rubber-soled slippers to knock them free with a wooden chair leg or broom handle (see fig, p.64)

3 Check breathing and pulse. Begin emergency cardiopulmonary resuscitation (see pp.233–6)

4 With cold water, treat the burns where electricity entered and left the body. Place in the recovery position (see pp.236–7) and call 999

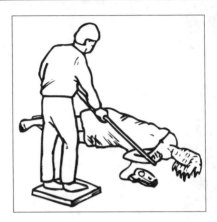

DANGER!

If electrocution is caused by a high-voltage source like overhead electricity cables, it will normally be fatal. DO NOT attempt to approach the victim to cut them off from the current source — high-voltage electricity can 'arc', or jump across a gap of up to 18 metres

Electric Shock And Electrocution
• •

An electric shock happens when someone touches a live wire or an appliance or any part of it which has become live, i.e. has an electric current flowing through it. It is terrifying to deal with, whether it happens to yourself or someone else. Most electric shocks in the home are not fatal although in wet conditions, such as in a bathroom, fatalities are more likely to happen. But it is important that you know what to do in advance in case you are faced with a case of electrocution. Page 63 details the measures to take should you ever be called on to cope with it.

The table of Electrocution Injuries on page 66 lists the commonest injuries you would have to deal with in an electrocution case. With the right first-aid knowledge you can minimise any damage and possibly even save a life, but to be able to function effectively in

ELECTROCUTION INJURIES

- **SHOCK** Keep the victim warm and quiet while you call for help
- **NO BREATHING** Apply mouth-to-mouth resuscitation (see p.230)
- **NO PULSE** Apply chest compression (see p.234)
- **BURNS** These may be deep in the tissues and not all visible
- **FALL INJURIES** The victim may injure themselves if knocked off their feet

an emergency you should read the information on how to treat these injuries *now*, before you really need to – the last thing you want to do in an emergency is stand flicking through this book. (See the Medical Emergencies chapter, p.225.)

Following the safety instructions on p.68 should also help you avoid electrocution.

Electrical Emergencies

Aside from the happily rare occurrences of electrocution, any malfunctioning of your domestic electrical appliances should be more in the nature of an inconvenience rather than a full-scale emergency. Nevertheless, any dealings with electricity, even of the most minor, everyday kind, should never be undertaken lightly.

Know the risks

Electricity is available to us everywhere literally at the flick of a switch, but it is vital in any home emergency or repair job not to cut corners in terms of time, equipment and money, or to be tempted to take it for granted. Slip-ups can be dangerous, but working on your electricity system is in theory relatively straightforward as long as you take your time, take care and understand completely what you are doing.

Working safely with electricity

- Make certain the electricity supply is off (see DANGER! box, p.69)

- Before you start work on a circuit, double-check it is disconnected by plugging in an appliance you know works; better still, use a circuit tester

- Use good-quality, British Standards-rated materials

- Be sure you are using correctly rated plugs, fuses, flexes and cables for the job (see pp.84 and 86)

- Always unplug an appliance before you try to work with it or repair it

- Never touch an electric appliance or fitting with wet hands or use an electric appliance in wet conditions

- If you feel at all uncertain, or that you are getting out of your depth, stop immediately and call an electrician

However, if you are at all uncertain about any aspect of domestic repair work involving electricity – even down to the minor-grade repairs which are among those described in this chapter – you may feel safer employing a professional, qualified electrician.

Before you begin any electrical repair work, a basic knowledge of how your domestic electricity system works will help you understand why things may have gone wrong, and what is the safest way to put them right.

DANGER!

NEVER work on the fixed wiring system without first switching off the electricity at the mains. As a double-failsafe, take with you the fuse of the circuit you are working on to make sure no-one else can re-connect the supply. Tell others in the house what you are doing, in any case

Your Wiring System

The electrical supply to your house comes
from the mains through the meter, the fuse
box and consumer unit (see below). From
there fused circuits carry electricity around
the house via the fixed wiring system – that
is, the sockets, switches, ceiling and wall
lights. One circuit serves each individual
system, including lighting, central heating
and heavy-duty items like cookers and

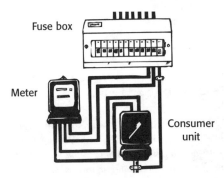

Fuse box

Meter

Consumer
unit

storage heaters. This arrangement allows you to turn off the power to any one circuit to make necessary repairs.

In the vast majority of cases nowadays, the circuits pass around the house in a ring which begins and ends at the consumer unit. If your wiring is of the older type and you do not have a consumer unit like the one illustrated, you should have your system checked and modernised by a qualified electrician.

Each circuit is protected by a fuse or circuit breaker. Newer types of circuit breakers are also fitted with residual current devices which shut off the power instantly if a disruption to the balance of live and neutral currents is detected anywhere on the circuit. In practice, this means that if your toddler sticks a knitting needle into a socket or you cut through the flex while using your electric lawn mower, the circuit will shut down automatically. Obviously, it is well worth investing in such a potential life-saver.

A faulty circuit

A fault on one of your domestic electricity
circuits should be relatively easy to spot,
especially if the individual circuits are
labelled on the consumer unit itself. All the
lights, or the storage heaters, or whatever is
served by that circuit, will cut out.

Discovering the fault

Fuses are safety valves on electricity circuits
and they blow for a reason. This can be:

- a fault in the balance of the current: live
  and neutral wires may be touching, or
  electricity may be leaking to earth
  through faulty wiring, a faulty appliance,
  tampering with sockets or a water
  spillage over the supply

- an overload of the system: too many
  heavy-duty appliances can demand a
  level of current which the circuit cannot
  cope with

Try to establish what could have caused the fuse to blow before you start any repair job. Did you switch on a certain appliance? If so, plug another appliance into that socket to test that the fault is really on the circuit and not with the appliance itself. Are there lots of big appliances being run off that circuit? You may need modifications to your circuitry to cope with larger demands. Replace the fuse in the suspect appliance, too, in case that has blown. Trial and error is really the only way to discover the cause and correct the fault.

Correcting the fault

Three types of fuses in consumer units govern most domestic electricity circuits. Which type you have will depend largely on the age of the circuitry. They are:

- a circuit breaker (see p.71)
- a cartridge fuse
- a rewirable fuse

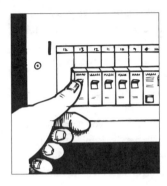

Resetting a switch-type circuit breaker

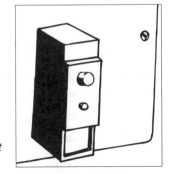

Simply press the button to reset this type of circuit breaker

Resetting a circuit breaker This is the easiest type of fuse repair to make. Simply switch it back on again, or press in the reset button.

Mending a cartridge fuse This type of fuse is housed in a little plug which you pull out of its socket on the consumer unit. Inside you will see the fuse cartridge which normally shows no sign of having blown. Take it out and replace it with a new one, snapping it into place between the metal grips, as you would a fuse cartridge on a plug. Make sure

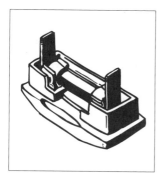

A cartridge fuse is similar to any fuse you would find in a plug

the new fuse you put in is of the rating
recommended on the fusebox.

If the fuses on the consumer unit are not
labelled and you don't know which one
relates to which circuit, you will have to try
each one methodically. As you go, it is
worthwhile to write above each fuse the name
of the circuit it controls. This will save you
having to repeat the exercise in the future
should another fuse need repaired.

Mending a rewirable fuse With this type of
fuse you will see instantly where the fault lies
– its wire, which is visible inside its casing,
will have snapped or melted. In this case,
undo the terminal screws retaining the old
wire, take it out (noting how it is threaded)
and replace it with another of the correct
rating. Cut off any extra wire projecting
beyond the terminal screws.

If the fuse blows again after you have gone
through all these steps, don't keep trying –
it's time to call in a qualified electrician.

Undoing the screw terminals of a rewirable fuse

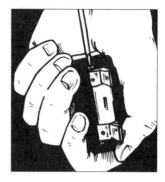

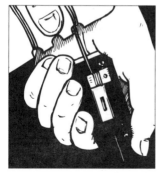

Replacing with the new fuse wire

Plugs, Fuses And Flexes

The electric current running through the circuits of your domestic fixed wiring system flows through plugs, fuses and flexes to power your domestic appliances. It is as important as for the fixed wiring system that safety rules and advice for these three items are followed to the letter – by doing this you keep yourself and your family as safe as a properly functioning system allows.

Plugs

Plugs, of course, form the vital safety link between the electricity current and the appliance wiring. Almost all appliances for sale nowadays come pre-fitted with moulded plastic plugs, relieving you of the chore of fitting one, but you may well still have to change a plug on an older appliance. This is how to do it.

1. To connect a new flex, cut back the white flex sheath with a knife or wire strippers. The sheath fits under the cable-grip bar at the bottom of the plug.

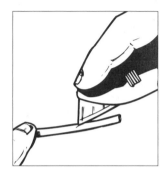

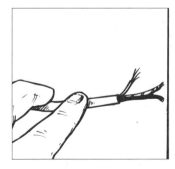

2. Strip away 12 mm of the coloured sheath of the copper core wires. Twist the wires together.

3. Connect up the cores to the terminals (see below), snap in the fuse, re-check the connections and cable grip, then screw shut the cover again.

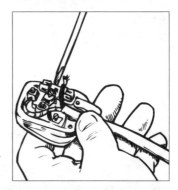

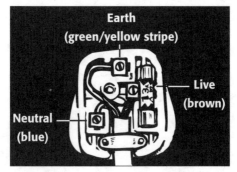

Earth
(green/yellow stripe)

Live
(brown)

Neutral
(blue)

DANGER!

It is vital that you connect up the wires properly when wiring a plug. Take the time to make doubly sure this simple task is done properly by always double-checking before you close the plug that the wires are in the right place. If the live (brown-covered) wire is not connected to the fuse, you could be running the risk of electrocution.

Fuses

The plug also carries a fuse cartridge which is linked to the live wire. It operates in the same way, although on a smaller scale, as a fuse in the main fusebox and forms part of your protection against electrocution by a malfunction in the plug or appliance. It is vital, to protect the equipment and those who use it, that the right fuse is used with each appliance.

The sign that a fuse on an appliance has blown is if the appliance cuts out and will not work when plugged into another socket on a different circuit. Take the plug apart to replace the fuse. Check that the new fuse you are fitting is of the correct rating for the appliance – this will be stamped somewhere on the appliance. Don't just assume it's right and fit the same one as you remove, as it may have been wrong in the first place.

The illustration opposite shows how to change a fuse.

DANGER!

NEVER use an incorrectly rated fuse on an appliance for which it was not recommended. Fitting a 13-amp fuse will allow any appliance to run, but a power surge would put your appliance at risk and might even cause a fire. NEVER EVER use a plug without a fuse – it is your safeguard against electrocution. Without it you could be risking your and your family's lives.

Lever the old fuse out with a screwdriver and replace it with a correctly rated one for the appliance it serves.

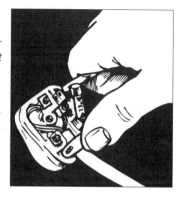

The tables on the following page offer a guide to recommended amp ratings. Remember, these are intended only as a rough guide. Check your particular appliance's rating plate for the wattage (marked W); alternatively, look in the handbook to find the recommended amp rating of the fuse. If you don't have the appliance handbook any more, ask a qualified electrician.

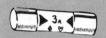

**3-AMP FUSES:
UP TO 720 WATTS**

Blender

Clock

Computer

DIY tools (some)

Electric blanket

Extractor

Food processor

Free-standing lamp

Freezer

Fridge

Hairdryer

Hi-fi

Radio/tape player

TV & VCR

**13-AMP FUSES:
OVER 720 WATTS**

Deep-fat fryer

Dishwasher

DIY tools (some)

Electric heater

Electric kettle

Fan heater

Lawn mower

Microwave

Oven

Toaster

Tumble dryer

Vacuum cleaner

Washing machine

Flexes

The flex is the means by which electricity
flows from the plug into your appliance.
Through it, electricity flows along the live
wire (in the brown-coloured insulating
sheath) to whatever appliance is being
powered, back through the neutral wire (in
the blue sheath). Most appliances also have a
third, earth wire (in the green-and-yellow-
striped sheath) which lets the electricity pass
to the socket.

You will need a new flex for an appliance
as soon as the old one shows any signs of
wearing – don't wait until the coloured wires
are showing through.

Different types and sizes of flexes are
needed for different jobs. While the flex on
your appliance at present can be used as an
indicator, don't always assume that it's right.
Double-check on suitability with the
hardware dealer when you are buying a
replacement.

THE RIGHT FLEX FOR THE JOB

APPLIANCES	FLEX TYPE
Double-insulated appliances (stamped ☐ e.g. TVs)	2-core
Electric heaters	Braided
Irons, kettles	Unkinkable
Hanging lights	Heat-resistant
Most other appliances	Normal

Extending a flex

If you need a longer flex, the safest and most efficient option is to remove the old flex completely and fit a new one of the right length. To make a temporary extension, however, you must use a flex connector. Never extend a flex simply by taping the two sets of wires together with insulating tape – it could be pulled apart if someone trips over it, or overheat and cause a fire.

The coloured wires are paired at the terminals – blue to blue, brown to brown and green and yellow together in the middle. See also DANGER! box below.

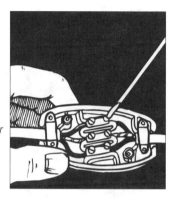

DANGER!

If you fit a temporary flex extension, you must ensure that the socket fitting (female part) is connected to the mains and the plug (male part) connected to the appliance. To fit them the other way would be to leave the exposed pins with a live current flowing through them. See p. 88

The illustration below shows the correct
orientation of male and female fittings in a
flex extension.

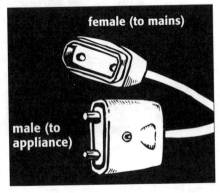

Flex extensions used outdoors If you have a
large garden or do outdoor DIY work you
may find yourself with too short a length of
flex to reach the power source. The moulded
electrical fittings which commonly protect
electrical appliances nowadays may make it

impossible for you to replace the flex with a
longer one, certainly without returning the
item to the manufacturer. Consequently, you
may find that you have to use flex extensions
in these cases.

A simple safety tip when working outdoors
is to wrap the connection in a polythene bag
taped into place. That way, if you
accidentally tug the connection loose, you
don't run the risk of an electric shock from
the moisture in the air or ground.

The table below shows the Don'ts and Dos
of flex safety.

> ✗ Don't ever pull out plugs by tugging the flex
> ✗ Don't run flexes under carpets
> ✗ Don't ever extend a flex without a proper
>   connector properly fitted
> ✔ Do keep flexes as short as possible
> ✔ Do keep flexes away from heat sources
>   such as fires and hobs
> ✔ Do regularly check the condition of flexes

Adaptors and extension leads

'One appliance, one socket' is the golden rule and you should avoid using adaptors at all costs. They overload sockets in two ways:

- an electrically overloaded socket can overheat and catch fire
- an adaptor with several plugs can be partly pulled down out of the socket by their weight, exposing live pins and endangering anyone touching it

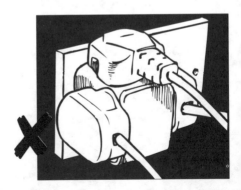

Anyone who needs to use adaptors needs more sockets – doubles installed where singles exist at present, or spurs coming off the circuit. These are not major jobs for a qualified electrician.

In the short term, if an electrician cannot do the work for you immediately, a multi-socket extension lead like the one shown below, is a far better option than an adaptor.

The table on the next page shows some Don'ts and Dos of multi-socket adaptor use.

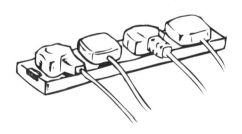

✗ Don't use an extension lead showing any
signs of overheating, at sockets, plug or flex

✔ Do keep the extension lead flex uncoiled to
avoid its overheating

✔ Do note the wattage of appliances run off
the extension lead to ensure the load stays
within the wall-socket's 3000-watt maximum
capacity

Light Fittings

The tired old jokes about changing lightbulbs
may come to mind as you scan the next few
paragraphs, but even in something as
commonplace as lightbulb-changing there is
always a first time for someone somewhere –
not to mention some safety rules to observe.

And unlike standard lightbulbs, fluorescent
lights can last for anything up to six years or
beyond. Changing them is therefore a less
familiar job, but the steps are just as easy to
follow.

Changing a lightbulb

It will be fairly obvious even to the uninitiated when a lightbulb has blown. Nine times out of ten it will happen as you turn the light on, when the initial surge of power will find out any weakness existing in the fitting. An instantaneous flash precedes the 'pop' of the filament breaking inside the bulb before the light goes out again.

There are two basic types of tungsten-filament lightbulbs:

- bayonet fitting
- screw fitting

Check which type you need before buying a replacement. You will also need to check the maximum wattage recommended for the light. Most lights nowadays take 60-watt bulbs, although the rating can be lower or higher. Do not exceed wattage recommended on your lamp: you risk overheating the shade.

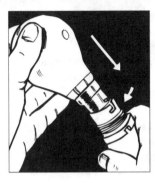

Bayonet fitting: Remove the old bulb by pushing it down and twisting it anticlockwise to free the pins. To fit the new bulb, simply reverse the process.

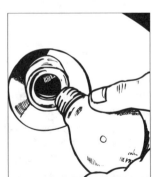

Screw-fitting bulb

Screw-fitting lightbulbs are becoming increasingly common, especially on 'feature' and display lighting.

And although tungsten-halogen bulbs look different in operation from normal tungsten bulbs, they still share the same types of fitting.

As always, before you begin any electrical work, disconnect the appliance you are about to work on: unplug the light from the socket, or switch a fixed light off at the wall.

Changing a fluorescent fitting

Unlike a normal lightbulb, an old fluorescent light will warn you, usually by flickering, not lighting properly, or discolouring at the ends, that the tube needs to be replaced.

There are three types of tube fittings:

- bayonet fitting
- two-pin fitting
- circular fitting

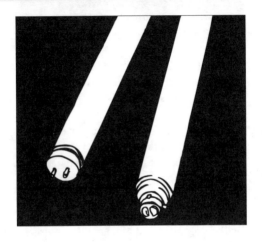

Like a bayonet fitting on a lightbulb (see p. 94), a fluorescent tube twists out of its holders, while the two-pin version is spring-loaded (see the illustration above) and simply pushed into place. A circular tube has pins which plug into a socket on the fixture.

If, however, the tube has been replaced relatively recently, the problem may not lie

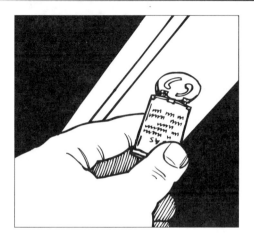

with the tube itself but with the starter
(shown above), the automatic switch that
fires the tube to light. Modern rapid-start
lights do not use starters, but many older
types do. Starters, which are usually found
protruding slightly from the casing of the
light also have a bayonet fitting. To remove a
starter, simply twist it through 45 degrees

anticlockwise and pull it clear.

Take a note of the fitting and wattage of the tube when you go to buy a replacement, or take the starter with you, as each new fitting needs to be identical to the one it's replacing.

5 Water

Be Prepared!

For most major plumbing emergencies, you need one basic piece of information: the location of the stopcocks and valves to shut off the supply of water coming into your house.

The best time to find this is not as water floods down the walls soaking the carpets and furnishings, so it is worth making the effort to find it now.

Turning off the water

At the main stopcock

In a full-scale emergency such as a burst pipe, the most direct action is to turn off the water completely at the main stopcock – know its location.

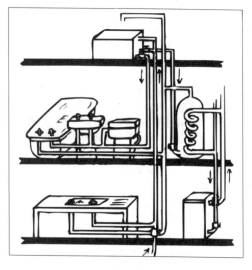

The arrangement of a typical domestic plumbing system

The main stopcock is normally found:

- under the kitchen sink
- in the utility room
- in the airing cupboard
- in the basement

The kitchen tap is usually the only tap fed directly from the main; from there, the water passes on to fill the cold-water tank, usually in the loft. The rest of the house is supplied from there.

In some older houses, all the taps are fed directly off the main and often have their own stopvalves, but in emergencies, you should simply turn off the main stopcock.

At the outside stopcock

If you cannot turn off the water using the main stopcock, you can in an emergency shut off the supply at the outdoor stopcock. This belongs to your water supplier, and is set up to 1 metre into the ground, either on the pavement outside the house or just inside your property boundary.

The main problem with this option is that you may have to be reasonably well organised, with your own key to fit the stopcock. You can buy these from DIY or plumbers' suppliers. Find out first if the stopcock has a cross-head mechanism or a notch mechanism.

Individual pipes and taps

The pipes from the cold-water tank usually have their own gate valves. This allows you to shut off water to a particular pipe for minor repairs, leaving the supply to the rest of the house unaffected.

But some pipes may have no gate valve. To shut off the water supply to these, you will have to drain the tank. Do this by turning off the water at the main stopcock, then turning on the cold taps to drain the tank.

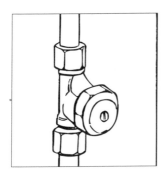

*Gate valve on
a pipe*

Frozen Pipes

The first sign you may have of a frozen pipe
is when no water will run out of a cold tap.
The tap, or cistern, which will not work
normally is the one whose pipe is affected and
the most likely place to look for the freeze-up
is in the loft. Improvements in insulation,
shutting heat out of the loft and keeping it in
the house, mean pipes are more liable to
freeze there than anywhere else in the house.

ACTION!

DEALING WITH A FROZEN PIPE

1 If the pipe has frozen and has obviously burst, turn off the water supply to it

2 Check for any cracks before you start

3 Carefully thaw the pipe with gentle heat from a source such as a hairdryer or a fan heater. Do not leave the heat source unattended

4 Play the heat along the parts most likely to be frozen – unlagged pipes and bends

5 If there is a crack in the pipe, slow thawing will minimise any risk of a large burst

6 Repair the crack (see p.105)

Once you have unfrozen your pipe, you can follow the same procedure for repairing it as you would for any burst pipe.

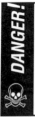

If any part of the hot-water system seems to be frozen or blocked, turn off the boiler immediately. A blockage in either the system or in the pipes leading into it will overheat the system, carrying the risk of an explosion in the boiler

Burst Pipes

Unless you are an enthusiastic and competent plumbing DIY-er, you will probably want simply to repair the pipe temporarily to minimise any damage until a plumber arrives.

To begin, shut off the water to the pipe by closing the gate valve, drain it and let it dry.

> ## DANGER! ☠
>
> If water from a burst pipe has reached any light fitting or other electrical appliance, do not touch the fitting or any controlling switch. Instead, turn all electrical power off at the fuse box and call in an electrician immediately

What to use

Epoxy putty This is sold in a special kit with two separate tubes; once mixed they will start to harden and you will only have about 30 minutes to complete the repair. Epoxy putty will produce a reasonably strong bond, but the pipe will still need to be repaired eventually.

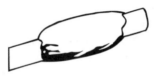

Epoxy putty repair

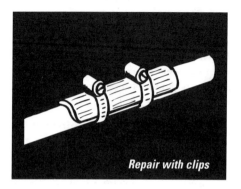

Repair with clips

Hose and hose clips More impromptu is a
piece of hose; a garden hose will do. Cut a
length long enough to extend 10 cm beyond
the damaged part, and slit it down the side so
you can slip it over the crack. Secure the pipe
with hose clips, or Jubilee clips. If you don't
have these, some pieces of wire twisted tight
with pliers should hold the hose in place.
Tape The simplest way to hold together a
crack is simply to bind it with waterproof
repair tape to hold it until a plumber arrives.

Protection from bursts

One burst and the disruption – and damage –
it can cause will be enough to convince you
never to repeat the experience. There are steps
you can take to lessen the chances of a repeat.

How to avoid burst pipes

- Lag the pipes. Several materials are
  available; choose the best for you

- Insulate the cold-water tank. Again,
  there is a range of products on offer

- Do not extend roof insulation under
  the cold-water tank. Heat from the
  room below will help avoid freeze-ups

- In cold weather, keep the central
  heating ticking over at a low level,
  especially at night or if you are going
  away for a time. It is less distressing to
  pay for the extra fuel than to return to
  a flooded house

Blocked Pipes

Less dramatically damaging than burst pipes,
waste-pipe blockages can be an inconvenience
at best, and downright messy at worst.

Sink and bath blockages

The easiest time to tackle a blockage is when
the water first seems to be slow in draining –
try not to put off the job until the pipe blocks
completely.

Blockages are usually caused by a build-up
of debris, such as food, paper, hair, fat or tea
leaves, which has fallen down the plughole
and gathered, usually in the trap under the
sink. (The trap is the U-bend or other shaped
bend in the pipe where water collects to seal
off the sink from the entrance to the waste
system.)

There are several ways to treat blockages,
at this early stage and when they totally bung
up the pipe.

Plunger

The most straightforward option and the one most people will try first. A plunger can be used for a partial or a complete blockage. Different types of plunger are available; all work by creating a suction to dislodge the blockage.

- the modern plastic compression type of plunger is filled with water, held in place over the plughole and then pumped up and down (see below)

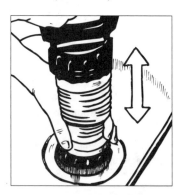

- the older rubber suction type is also worked with a pumping action
- any thick material, such as a springy cloth, soft ball or sponge, which can cover the plughole

Remember to block up the overflow with some cloth or a rag, and keep enough water in the sink to cover the plunger cup.

Drain clearer

This is sold at supermarkets and ironmongers. It is poured down the sink and contains corrosives which help dissolve the blockage.

DANGER!

Drain clearers contain corrosives to dissolve blockages – these also dissolve human tissue, so wear protective clothing and eyewear, and follow pack instructions to the letter. Be especially careful if you try to clear the trap after unsuccessfully using a drain clearer

Drain clearers should only be used at the
partial-block stage, not when the sink or bath
is totally blocked and full of water.

A greener and safer alternative is to make
your own. Mix 100 g baking soda with 200
ml vinegar in 1 litre of boiling water. Cover it
and let it sit for a minute, then pour it down
the drain. Leave it overnight and rinse the
drain thoroughly with hot water next morning.

Clearing the trap

The under-sink trap is the most likely blockage
site. It is normally attached with connecting
nuts to the pipes which take the water out to
the waste system.

Older U-bend traps may have a removable
drain plug; alternatively, you may have to
take off the complete trap section. With
modern 'bottle' traps, you should be able to
unscrew the whole base section to clean it out.
You must be very careful if you have already
unsuccessfully used a caustic drain clearer.

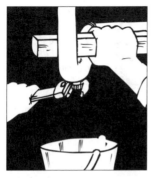

U-bend Traps
1. Put a bucket below to catch any debris or water.
2. Unscrew the drain plug with a spanner or wrench.
3. With your other hand, hold a piece of wood in the U-bend to keep the pipe steady.

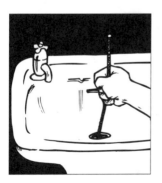

4. Push a piece of net curtain wire or a similar flexible or bendy wire down the plughole.
5. Wiggle it around to push the debris out of the drain plug.

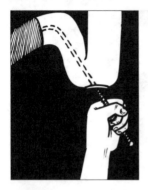

6. If the blockage is still intact, push the wire along the other section of the pipe to clear out any block from there.
7. Try to pull the debris out towards you; pushing it into the pipe may make it stick further down.

If the pipe has no drain plug, unscrew the trap section.

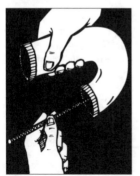

1. Unscrew the connecting nuts with a wrench.
2. Wiggle the trap until it comes away from the pipes.
3. Clear it out with wire and replace.

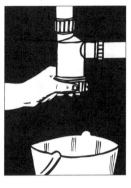

Bottle Traps
1. Put a bucket under the trap to catch any debris and water that comes out.
2. Unscrew the bottom section of the bottle trap.

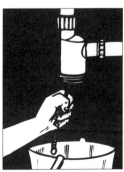

3. Push a piece of net curtain wire or a similar bendy wire up the pipe towards the sink and along the waste pipe to dislodge the block.

Protection from pipe blockages

It is a relatively easy job to maintain your domestic plumbing system in good order and guard against blockages. Following the straightforward practices listed on the page opposite can help. Remember that the basic rule for clear drains is – don't let anything float down the plughole.

Toilet Blockages

As with pipe blockages, blockages in the toilet are best tackled at the first sign of trouble. They call for special tools and clearing any blockage can be messy and smelly work, so you may prefer to call in a plumber.

Below are remedial cures which may relieve the blockage, at least in the short term. Always wear rubber gloves when working at the toilet.

How to avoid blocked pipes

- Never pour fat down the sink, either with or without hot water; even a little gums up the pipes and can give other debris a sticky surface to cling to. Instead, let it cool, seal it in a plastic bag and bin it.

- Do not let hair, tea leaves, vegetable scrapings or other material float down the drain. An inexpensive trap fitted over the plughole can catch any debris.

- This simple, eco-friendly mix, used weekly, will keep household pipes clear: mix 50g salt, 50 g baking soda and 25 g cream of tartar. Pour it down the drain, then pour down a pint of boiling water, followed by a pint of cold water.

Cleaning the bend

If you know the blockage in your toilet is just beyond the bend, try pushing down a flexible net-curtain wire or a thick wire bent into a hook-shape at the end. Bail out the water from the pan before you begin, to give you easier access to the bend.

Water force

A low-tech option known to work, but which carries its own risks, is to stand above the toilet on a secure set of steps and pour a bucket of water in from on high. The force of the water may just help dislodge any minor blockage. A stout heart and steady eye are needed – and remember to keep an eye on the water-level in the bowl.

Plunger

As with sink blockages, a plunger will clear a blockage in a toilet waste pipe. But a much

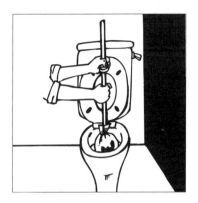

bigger one is needed for this job, and you will probably have to hire one from a tool-hire shop.

You could also try making your own (as shown above): wrap a plastic bag around the head of an old mop and secure it tightly with string. After bailing out some of the water, pump the plunger carefully but vigorously up and down in the toilet pan.

Protection from toilet blockages

Remembering a few straightforward rules will help ensure your toilet stays working well.

How to avoid a blocked toilet

FOLLOW THE SIMPLE RULE:
ONLY PUT DOWN THE TOILET WHAT IS MEANT TO GO DOWN IT!

● Never put cotton wool, cotton buds, nappies or kitchen paper down the toilet – all are big blockage-causers. Keep a bin in the loo for such items

● Wrap and bin all sanitary products: although most are small and soluble, they still block pipes, and there are problems in their treatment at sewage works

● Be careful what foods you throw down the toilet: tea-leaves are OK (although better wrapped in paper and binned), but avoid bigger items

Everyday Problems

Dripping tap

If a tap drips after you turn it off, and there is a little 'give' in its on/off action, it probably needs a new washer. While hardly qualifying as an emergency, a dripping tap should be mended promptly. If the job is put off the sink or bath will stain, the washer will eventually split and the tap may unexpectedly jam on.

There is a range of tap types, but the basic steps in changing washers are the same. They come in different sizes; these are generally:

- 12 mm for sinks
- 19 mm for baths

However, they can vary. If in doubt, buy several sizes – they cost pennies, and having a selection to hand could save you having to take a tap apart more than once. And even if you don't have the exact size, a larger washer can often be cut down to do the job.

Pillar and shrouded-head taps

These are the two main types of tap. Although dismantled in different ways, the method of changing the washer on each is the same.

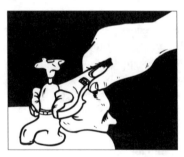

1. Turn off the water supply to the tap (see p.102) then turn the tap on to drain completely.

2. When no more water comes out, put the plug in the plughole to stop screws or other items falling in.

3A. For a pillar tap, unscrew the cover, by hand if possible. (If it is too stiff, put a cloth around the tap to protect it, then loosen it with a spanner.) Lift the cover to let you get at the headgear nut.

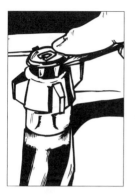

3B. For a shrouded-head tap, prise up the little 'H' or 'C' disk in the centre; this may reveal a central screw which is loosened to allow the tap head to pull off. Alternatively, it may pull straight off, or screw off as if you were continuing to turn off the tap.

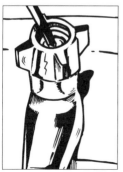

4. On both tap types, unscrew the headgear nut until the headgear can lift away. The washer is fixed to the jumper inside the tap. With some taps the jumper and washer will come away at the bottom of the headgear; in others, they will be left inside the tap.

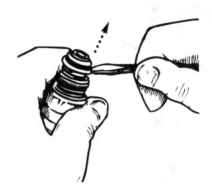

5. Remove the washer, either by prising it off the little button fixing it to the jumper, or unscrewing its fixing nut with a spanner and a pair of pliers. (You may need to use WD40 to loosen this nut, but if it is totally resistant a new jumper and washer together can be fitted.)

6. Fit the new washer and reassemble the tap. Remember to turn the tap off before turning the water supply back on.

Supataps (Reverse-pressure taps)

You do not need to turn off the water to change a washer on this tap; its internal valve gradually shuts off the water automatically as you loosen the nozzle.

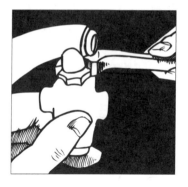

1. Loosen the nut above the nozzle then unscrew the nozzle anticlockwise (its screw mechanism works in reverse).

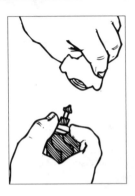

2. Tap the nozzle against something firm, e.g. a vinyl floor, or push a pencil or straw up inside it to push out the anti-splash unit which controls the water flow. The washer unit is on the end of it.

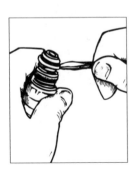

3. Pull out the old washer unit; you may need to use a screwdriver to prise it off.

4. Fit the new washer unit, then reassemble the tap following the same steps as before, in reverse order.

Mixer (Swivel nozzle) taps

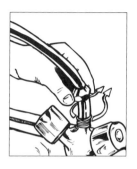

There is no need to cut off the water when repairing this tap.

1. Unscrew the shroud at the bottom of the tap. This will reveal a C-shaped circlip which holds the tap in place. Lever the circlip off, then remove the spout.

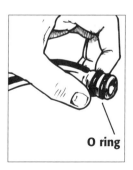

O ring

2. Take the old 'O' ring off and replace it with a new one of the same size. Reassemble the tap.

(On some older taps you will find the O ring inside the base of the tap, rather than on the spout.)

Nail hammered through a pipe

It is all too easy to pierce a pipe while you are fixing loose floorboards or laying a carpet.

You may instantly hear the water hissing out, but generally the first sign is a damp-related problem in the floor later or, if you have been working in an upstairs room, a damp patch on the ceiling of the room below.

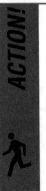

ACTION!

DEALING WITH A NAILED PIPE

1 Resist the urge to pull out the nail straight away; it will keep the flow at a moderate level

2 Shut off the water to the pipe and drain it by turning on the tap it feeds

3 Repair the leak temporarily (see pp.105–7) or call a plumber straight away for a permanent repair

If you are nailing down lots of damaged floorboards or laying a carpet, it is worth lifting some of the boards to check exactly where the pipes are; chalking their location on the floor will let you hammer around them in safety.

Cold central-heating radiators

Central-heating problems are for the most part beyond the scope of all but the most competent and confident DIY-er, and of this book. Central-heating systems are costly and relatively complicated, and as such are best left to professionals.

But one of the commonest central-heating faults can also, conveniently, be one of the easiest to deal with. The problem of radiators which are cold, or cold around the top, when they should be hot is generally a sign of air or gas having collected inside which is preventing the hot water flowing properly through and heating the system.

To bleed the radiator you will need a square-ended radiator key. These are supplied with your system, and they can also be bought at DIY stores or ironmongers.

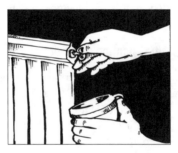

1. Holding a container or absorbent cloth under the radiator valve, turn the key to unscrew the valve one-quarter or -half turn at a time, until the air starts to hiss out.

2. When all the air has escaped, water will start to trickle out onto your cloth. Close the valve.

NOTE: If your radiators need to be bled regularly, and especially if you notice a gas smell as you bleed them, there may be corrosion in the system. Tackling it will be a job for an experienced professional.

6 Infestation

Don't Panic!

Few things in the home are guaranteed to cause a householder such instantaneous horror as the thought of playing host to an infestation. Most of us can live, albeit uneasily, with the thought of the microscopic insects and parasites that live, unseen, in and around the house, but when uninvited visitors are revealed in all their ugliness, many people (and not just the more delicate of us) want to run for the hills.

Unfortunately, there is also the added stigma that the presence of bugs reflects in some way on the cleanliness of your home. This is an outdated idea well past its use-by date. A new infestation reflects not at all on your domestic hygiene and, ironically, the cleaner your place is, the more attractive it becomes for many pests.

Many unwelcome domestic visitors are indeed dirty and a health hazard; some are parasitic, some merely unpleasant to look at; and some are just downright pests, but in any case you will want to be rid of them. And the speed of elimination is a far more accurate reflection of the standards of cleanliness in your home than their presence in the first place.

Of course, your particular infestation problem may not be of the insect variety – any visitors who are both uninvited and unwelcome must be regarded as pests. Into this category may fall rodents, wild animals, birds and even neighbourhood domestic animals. You may find any of these coming into your garden or your home in search of ready food and shelter. The information in this chapter will help you deal with all the main domestic infestation problems.

ACTION!

10 STEPS TO MAKE YOUR HOME LESS INVITING TO PESTS

1 Don't let dust and fluff lie

2 Use a good-quality vacuum with a hypo-allergenic filter

3 Move furniture as you clean

4 Clean up food scraps instantly

5 Empty household rubbish daily and keep outside bins tight shut

6 Keep unused food in the fridge or covered if it can't be chilled

7 Fit insect screens to regularly open windows, and to outer doors in summer

8 Seal gaps under doors, and around windows, pipes, cables

9 Check both loft and cupboards monthly for infestations

10 Only put out scraps for birds on tables or in feeders

Pest Control Options

You have a choice of approaches once you discover pests on your property – to let the local authority deal with it, to hire a private company to deal with it, or to deal with it yourself.

Public: local councils

Despite their ever-increasing financial constraints, local councils are still obliged to deal with any pests in your home which may be considered a threat to public health.

The services offered vary widely from one area to another, but the ones they will treat will probably include the following:

- vermin such as rats and mice
- stinging or biting insects such as wasps and fleas
- insects hazardous to public health such as cockroaches and lice

Some, but not all, of these pest-control services may be free; you can find out which by calling your local Environmental Health Department. Find its number under the entry for your local council in the phone book. If you are unemployed, are on income support or are a senior citizen you may be entitled to any of these services free of charge.

When deciding on your eradication programme, you may choose to make the Environmental Health Department your first port of call. Explain your problem and decide how to proceed on the basis of information coming back from them – it might be preferable to wait an extra two days to have the wasps' nest in your loft eradicated free of charge. It is also worth remembering that your problem may need more than one treatment. And explaining your special circumstances, such as a baby in the house, may qualify you to go to the head of the queue. There's no harm in trying!

Private: professional companies

Many private companies can take on the task of eradicating infestations from your home. But before you reach for the Yellow Pages, contact the British Pest Control Association (01332-294288), an industry body that gives information and advises on reputable firms who conform to their code of practice. As some of the chemicals and insecticides pest-control companies rely on are likely to be harmful to you if used incorrectly, you will need the reassurance of a reputable company – this is not a job to give corner-cutting cowboys.

The information you get back from your local Environmental Health Department may prompt you ultimately to decide to hire a private firm. You may also feel happier with the convenience and accountability that such firms can offer. Try to get quotes from more than one company so that you can compare the service offered as well as the cost.

Doing it yourself

You may decide to tackle the infestation yourself – and for some problems, such as head lice, you will have to.

Some larger-scale problems can still be dealt with on a DIY basis, but bear in mind that others do call for specialist knowledge, so you may find yourself having to do some swotting up on methods of eradication. This chapter will help point you in the right direction. You may also need protective gear, which you may be able to hire, but if your pest problem is best treated by chemicals not on sale to the general public, it may be time to call in the professionals. It is also worth remembering that if you do try to solve the problem yourself and get it wrong, you may in fact make the original problem worse.

But there is always preventative and remedial action you can take to reduce your chances of an infestation or, where one has occurred, to make sure that it doesn't happen twice.

DIY bug-busting: safety rules to follow

Whether you are treating a full-scale bug infestation or just spraying a can of Raid to zap a bluebottle, remember that you are using **poisons**: they are highly effective, but insects are not the only things that can be damaged by them. No pesticide can ever be regarded as safe. Keep yourself and your family safe – use them carefully and correctly.

DANGER!

- Follow the instructions to the letter
- Use a face mask and rubber gloves while you spray
- Remove or cover food
- After it has done its work, wash down any surface the pesticide fell on
- Keep children and pets away until the sprayed area is washed and dried
- Always store pesticides in their original containers and don't use these for any other purpose

Advantages of the three approaches

The local council offers:

- services that may be free
- paid services sometimes cheaper than the equivalent private cost

Private firms offer:

- a potentially quicker response time, especially at peak times like summer
- a wider range of eradication services than those of local councils

DIY remedies offer:

- potentially the fastest response time
- convenience and privacy
- a cheaper solution to some potentially costly pest problems

Types Of Infestation:
Insects And Animals By A–Z
• •

The following pages deal with individual pests, the dangers they present and how best to eradicate them.

Infestations are arranged in two groups. Pages 141–157 deal with insect infestations, but also pests such as ticks, which you may encounter outdoors and which can present a very real danger to your long-term health.

Pages 158–165 tackle larger pests such as rodents, which may invade your home, and uninvited garden visitors in the form of domestic and wild animals.

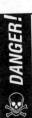

DANGER!

ALWAYS REMEMBER
Use and store pesticides and pest-control products ONLY where children and pets cannot possibly reach them

ANTS   [INSECTS; 3–5mm]

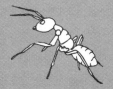

ASSOCIATED PROBLEMS:
- few from British garden ant
- in hot countries, pharaoh's ants and other species are dirty and dangerous

ATTRACTED TO:
- sweet smells

TREATMENTS:
- commercial deterrents, used to keep the ants out of your house; insecticides, to kill them, are only really effective if used on the nest. Both are widely available

OTHER COMMENTS:
- the traditional trick of pouring boiling water into the nest still has supporters but is probably of limited use without a follow-up dose of insecticide

BEDBUGS [INSECTS; 3–4mm]

ASSOCIATED PROBLEMS:
- bedbugs feed on human blood and their bites leave an itchy lump
- contamination of cracks in wallpaper and crevices in mattress and bedding

ATTRACTED TO:
- ready supplies of blood, usually in beds but sometimes in chairs and sofas

TREATMENTS:
- normally insecticide treatment, carried out by local council or private contractors

OTHER COMMENTS:
- bedbugs are difficult to spot as they only emerge in darkness
- they are now rare in this country but can remain dormant for up to 2 years

BEES   [INSECTS; up to 20mm]

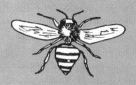

ASSOCIATED PROBLEMS:
- a swarm may enter a house en masse
- may sting if provoked; don't try to tackle a swarm yourself

TREATMENTS:
- contact the police or local council; local registered beekeepers should be able to collect a swarm for you

OTHER COMMENTS:
- some bees are protected by law and killing them is illegal

BOOK LICE [INSECTS; 1mm]

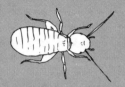

ASSOCIATED PROBLEMS:
- no associated health problems
- book lice damage and contaminate materials they feed on

ATTRACTED TO:
- moulds in damp book binding materials
- damp foodstuffs
- general damp conditions

TREATMENTS:
- treat infected areas with a dedicated booklice-killing insecticide
- ensure contaminated areas remain dry and well aired
- destroy any infected foodstuffs

CARPET BEETLES   [INSECTS; 2–4mm]

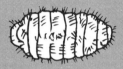

ASSOCIATED PROBLEMS:
- beetles eat holes into fabrics
- they carry human parasites

ATTRACTED TO:
- fabric with dried animal protein: wool, fur, leather
- dried-in foodstains on any fabric

TREATMENTS:
- vacuum well to remove beetles
- spray insecticide into skirting and floorboard cracks and under carpets
- clear lofts and eaves of old birds' nests
- dry-clean to kill beetles at all stages

OTHER COMMENTS:
- eggs are resilient; specialist advice may be needed to remove this tenacious pest

COCKROACHES [INSECTS; 10–24mm]

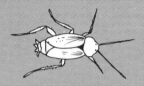

ASSOCIATED PROBLEMS:
- cockroaches spread bacteria when they walk and excrete
- they can cause serious food poisoning

ATTRACTED TO:
- warm, moist, dark places
- sewage and waste systems, drains and toilets

TREATMENTS:
- spray dedicated cockroach insecticide into the suspected source of infection

OTHER COMMENTS:
- roaches are persistent and will likely need professional treatment
- new waves may emerge 4-monthly and repeated treatments may be needed

FLEAS   [INSECTS; 2mm]

ASSOCIATED PROBLEMS:
- flea bites are itchy and irritating
- An out-of-control infestation can make a house almost uninhabitable

ATTRACTED TO:
- warm-blooded creatures
- cat, human, bird and dog fleas breed on those creatures but will bite any others

TREATMENTS:
- regular vacuuming
- remove old birds' nests from the loft
- spray flea killer into wall cracks
- treat infected pets with flea-killing preparations

FLIES [INSECTS; 3–12mm]

ASSOCIATED PROBLEMS:
- they spread parasitic worms and bacteria when they walk and excrete
- they can cause serious food poisoning
- some, such as clegs or horseflies, bite

ATTRACTED TO:
- fish and meat smells
- rotting organic rubbish

TREATMENTS:
- kill immediately with swatter or insecticide

OTHER COMMENTS:
- keep food covered and refrigerated
- keep flies away by strict hygiene and speedy disposal of rubbish
- spray outside bin with insecticide and keep it away from doors or windows

FLOUR BEETLES   [INSECTS; 3–4mm]

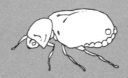

ASSOCIATED PROBLEMS:
● flour beetles contaminate flour, bread, biscuits, cereals, powdered soup and other dry foods
● no real associated health problems

ATTRACTED TO:
● dry foodstuffs in warm places

TREATMENTS:
● throw out infected food
● clear cupboard and apply insecticide for stored-product beetle control

OTHER COMMENTS:
● they may come via food or packaging that was badly kept in shop or storage
● they are not dirty but should be eradicated

HEAD LICE [INSECTS; 3mm]

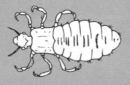

ASSOCIATED PROBLEMS:
- inflamed and itchy scalp
- can spread through entire household
- secondary skin infections from scratching

ATTRACTED TO:
- hair; clean hair is more attractive to them

TREATMENTS:
- remove lice, eggs (nits) and egg cases with a nit comb from the chemist's
- new non-toxic shampoo treatments are now coming on to the market

OTHER COMMENTS:
- There is concern about some shampoos which contain toxic organophosphates
- combs, brushes, bedding, towels and hats should be sprayed with insecticide

MITES   [ARACHNIDS; up to 2mm]

ASSOCIATED PROBLEMS:
- itch mite or scabies mite causes scabies by burrowing into the skin, usually on hands, causing an intensely itchy rash
- house dust mite's droppings may trigger asthma in allergy-prone people

ATTRACTED TO:
- a new host; itch mites are caught by close contact with a sufferer
- other mites, such as furniture and flour mites, are attracted by damp and moisture

TREATMENTS:
- prescription cream to kill itch mites
- ensure dry conditions and good ventilation to treat mites in the home
- apply mite insecticide to infested areas
- regular vacuuming (e.g. of mattresses)

MOSQUITOES [INSECTS; 3mm]

ASSOCIATED PROBLEMS:
- mosquito bites leave itchy swellings
- in tropical countries they carry malaria, yellow fever and other diseases

ATTRACTED TO:
- human blood, especially in the evening
- standing water, where they breed

TREATMENTS:
- swatting or fly-killer spray
- insect screens over doors and windows, or nets over beds
- spray or burn mosquito repellent
- drain away any still water outdoors

OTHER COMMENTS:
- Properties by a pool on warm-weather holidays can have mosquito problems

MOTHS   [INSECTS; 6–8mm]

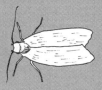

ASSOCIATED PROBLEMS:
- clothes moths cause damage to clothes, blankets, carpets and upholstery

ATTRACTED TO:
- natural fabrics, especially wool, but also fur, feathers, hair, cork, food scraps

TREATMENTS:
- make sure all clothes are clean, especially before storing them
- store clothes in sealed plastic bags
- use moth repellent in wardrobes and drawers; cedar, lavender and rosemary are good natural options

OTHER COMMENTS:
- the immature larvae, not the adult moths, eat their way into fabrics

SILVERFISH   [INSECTS; 12mm]

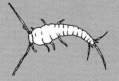

ASSOCIATED PROBLEMS:
- no apparent health risks

ATTRACTED TO:
- damp conditions in kitchens or bathrooms
- starchy food sources: glue, wallpaper paste, bookbinding, cereal-food crumbs

TREATMENTS:
- eliminate damp conditions
- seal up their food sources, such as high-carbohydrate foods
- kill with dedicated silverfish insecticide

TICKS   [ARACHNIDS; 1–2mm]

ASSOCIATED PROBLEMS:
- irritating or painful bites
- Lyme disease, a serious infection (mainly in Europe and north-east US)

ATTRACTED TO:
- birds, rodents, deer, dogs, humans

TREATMENTS:
- never try to pull a tick straight off: cover an attached tick with vaseline – the tick's bite will slacken enough to pull it off safely with tweezers
- for protection on country walks: cover limbs; use insect repellent with DEET (not on skin); check your and your child's body and clothes for ticks on return

WASPS [INSECTS; 10–15mm]

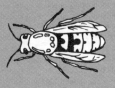

ASSOCIATED PROBLEMS:
- painful stings
- scavenging wasps can drag bacteria over surfaces they walk across

ATTRACTED TO:
- sweet food or drink

TREATMENTS:
- professional removal of wasps' nests; these are often unpredictable and shouldn't be handled by the public
- swatting or fly spray for individuals
- insect screens over doors and windows

OTHER COMMENTS:
- if you are stung, apply an anti-histamine
- wasp nuisance is worst in late summer
- if stings cause a reaction, get medical help

WOODWORM   [INSECTS; 3–6mm]

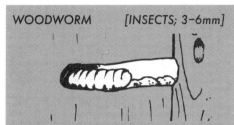

ASSOCIATED PROBLEMS:
- destructive boring of wood

ATTRACTED TO:
- any wood they come across

TREATMENTS:
- professional treatment, complete with guarantees, is best for large outbreaks
- isolate small, furniture-based outbreaks and treat with woodworm insecticide

OTHER COMMENTS:
- tell-tale 2mm holes on wood surface indicate woodworm; wood dust at the entrance means the outbreak is live
- woodworm may be in second-hand furniture – check for infestation; or they may fly in a window in late summer

BADGERS   [BIRDS & ANIMALS]

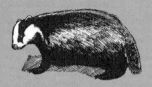

ASSOCIATED PROBLEMS:
- badgers' digging of vegetables and bulbs is destructive
- their dug-out latrines pit lawns

ATTRACTED TO:
- food: worms, insects, fruit, grain, acorns

DETERRENTS:
- approved repellent from garden centres
- chain-link fencing dug into the ground

OTHER COMMENTS:
- badgers have begun moving into suburban gardens in recent years
- it is illegal to injure or wilfully kill a badger or disturb their setts
- local badger groups may lend you low-voltage electric fences to deter them

BATS   [BIRDS & ANIMALS]

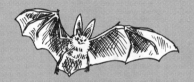

ASSOCIATED PROBLEMS:
- droppings are unsightly, though not dangerous, and may smell when wet
- bats may fly in through open windows

ATTRACTED TO:
- good roosting sites via holes less than 2 cm, especially at eaves and roof apex

DETERRENTS:
- there are no legal deterrants. It is illegal to kill, disturb or block the access of bats

OTHER COMMENTS:
- Bats do not damage buildings. For advice contact English Nature 01733-455000; Scottish Natural Heritage 0131-447 4784; Countryside Council for Wales 01248-370444

CATS　　　　　　　　[BIRDS & ANIMALS]

ASSOCIATED PROBLEMS:
- unpleasant urine smells in the garden
- excreting in garden gravel
- crushing fragile plants
- threat to garden birds and mammals

ATTRACTED TO:
- newly turned soil

TREATMENTS:
- sonic cat deterrents
- mothballs left around the garden

OTHER COMMENTS:
- cat and dog excrement carry parasites which are not just health hazards but endanger children and unborn babies. If you are able, clean up after your pet – take responsibility for your animal!

FOXES   [BIRDS & ANIMALS]

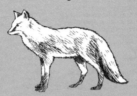

ASSOCIATED PROBLEMS:
- foxes dig holes on lawns
- scavenging at bins and bird tables

ATTRACTED TO:
- food: rabbits, birds, vermin, scraps

DETERRENTS:
- approved repellent from garden centres
- secure bins, raise bird-table heights,
  keep small outdoor pets securely caged
- low-voltage electric fences; see *Other
  comments* at Badgers, p. 158

OTHER COMMENTS:
- ever-adaptable foxes have moved into
  towns in the past 25 years. They eat
  vermin and many people welcome them
- it is illegal to poison or gas foxes

MICE [BIRDS & ANIMALS]

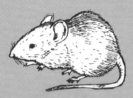

ASSOCIATED PROBLEMS:
- mice spread bacteria when they walk and excrete
- they can cause serious food poisoning
- their gnawing damages cables, pipes and even house structures

ATTRACTED TO:
- food sources
- warmth and shelter for nest sites

TREATMENTS:
- blocking up entry holes
- DIY or professional rodenticides
- baited mousetraps

OTHER COMMENTS:
- whole generations of mice can multiply in weeks and months, so act quickly

MOLES   [BIRDS & ANIMALS]

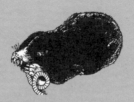

ASSOCIATED PROBLEMS:
- tunnels and hills damage lawns and young plant roots

ATTRACTED TO:
- sand- and clay-soil areas with plentiful food supply, i.e. worms and insects

DETERRENTS:
- sonic devices pushed into garden soil disperse moles humanely

OTHER COMMENTS:
- moles are a mixed blessing: their tunnelling can drain waterlogged soil, and they prey on harmful insect larvae

PIGEONS [BIRDS & ANIMALS]

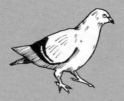

ASSOCIATED PROBLEMS:
- droppings damage buildings, cars and gardens
- droppings carry transmissible diseases
- mites cause skin disease in humans
- feather dust triggers allergic reactions

ATTRACTED TO:
- ready food supply
- easy nesting sites, e.g. under eaves

DETERRENTS:
- keep rubbish in secure bins
- seal potential nest sites with mesh wire

OTHER COMMENTS:
- the RSPB advises on pigeon-proofing your house (tel 01767-680551)

RATS   [BIRDS & ANIMALS]

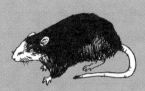

ASSOCIATED PROBLEMS:
- rats spread bacteria when they walk and excrete
- they spread and carry serious diseases
- their gnawing damages cables, pipes and even house structures

ATTRACTED TO:
- ready food supply
- easy nesting sites, e.g. sheds

TREATMENTS:
- DIY baits for individual sightings
- professionally used rodenticides

OTHER COMMENTS:
- keep children and pets away from affected areas and rodenticide baits
- protect baits from non-target wildlife

Common Pests: month-by-month guide

	Jan	Feb	Mar	Apr	May
Ants			○	○	○
Carpet beetles				○	●
Cockroaches	○	○	○	○	○
Fleas					○
Flies				○	○
Head lice	○	○	○	○	○
Mice	●	●	○	○	○
Mosquitoes				○	○
Rats	●	●	○	○	○
Wasps					
Woodworm					○

○ Active   ● Most active

Jun	Jul	Aug	Sep	Oct	Nov	Dec
○	●	○				
○		○	●			
○	○	○	○	○	○	○
○	○	○	●	●		
●	●	○	○			
○	○	○	○	○	○	○
○	○	○	○	○	●	●
○	○	○	○	○	○	
○	○	○	○	○	●	●
○	○	●	○	○		
○	●	○	○			

Other pests

Of course, in many other cases, pests are in the eye, or the attitude, of the beholder. Infestations in the home are never welcome, but people vary much more in their reaction to garden visitors. While many town-dwellers are delighted to catch sight of a fox in their garden, the reaction on a farm might not be so welcoming. And there is probably not much you will be able to do if a colony of magpies decides you have the best roosting tree in the neighbourhood. On the other hand, you can take action to protect yourself from a neighbour's unsecured dog roaming about.

If you are seriously concerned about a particular uninvited visitor to your garden or grounds, your first stop should be your environmental health department. They will be able to advise on your rights, responsibilities and what action that can be taken, if any, to exclude pests and intruders from your garden.

7 Rot, Damp & Climate Problems

Prevent Problems

Parasites and uninvited domestic visitors such as those described in Chapter 6 are bad enough, but damp-related problems, such as rot, are among the biggest threats to the fabric of your building.

As ever, prevention is better than cure. When you are buying a house, remember it may be a false economy to have a cheap survey done on the property. Be sure that the survey you choose will check for potential problems such as dry rot, in the unventilated areas where it is most likely to crop up. And if you are buying a new house, don't assume that it will therefore be immune from such problems. For example, wood which has been left outdoors to become soaking wet

can be, and often is, built into the framework
of new houses, and they may also be built on
previously waterlogged land which has been
inadequately drained and filled. Some new
house 'guarantees' are not worth the paper
they are written on, so be sure to arrange for a
full survey before you buy. And check *fully* –
with a lawyer if necessary – the builder's
obligations to put right any subsequent
problems, before you put your name to
anything.

A simple annual check will help maintain
your house in good condition, keeping you
warm and dry inside, and keeping out water,
your number one enemy. You may even think
it worthwhile to have your house professionally surveyed every two or three years.
Some mortgage lenders offer their clients just
such a house-check survey at a discounted
rate, so if an offer like this lands on your
doormat, don't dismiss it – you could be saving
yourself thousands of pounds in the long run.

ACTION!

KEEP YOUR HOME SAFE!
A YEARLY EXTERIOR CHECK-UP

1 With binoculars, check slates, ridges, valleys, eaves and any flat roofs

2 Check the loft for signs of leaks

3 Keep chimneys swept and well ventilated

4 Do a rainy-day check on gutters and drainpipes

5 Clear soil or debris from damp-proof courses (they should have 15 cm clearance) and airbricks

6 Check brickwork and mortar for cracks and splits

7 Check door and window fittings and paint; look out for draughts

8 Clear any moss or algae off walls and roofs

DANGER!

SAFE LARGE-SCALE ROT ERADICATION

- Use a company that does not use the toxic chemicals lindane, PCP or TBTO

- Move out during treatment, no matter how inconvenient

- Stay out at least 48 hours, and better still a week

- Keep all rooms ventilated afterwards

- Do not sleep in treated bedrooms for at least 7 nights

Dry Rot

Dry rot is guaranteed to fill householders with dread, at its potential for eating through both the fabric of a house and the finances of the owner. If you are unlucky enough to find it in your home, you *must* deal with it quickly – dry rot can spread frighteningly fast and, if left untreated, can ultimately damage a house beyond repair.

DRY ROT

CAUSES:
- indoor damp wood with poor ventilation and reasonable warmth

SIGNS:
- pungent, musty, mushroomy smell
- soft, silver cloud-like growths on wood; fruiting bodies surrounded by red spores are seen in advanced outbreaks
- wood turns dark brown

ASSOCIATED DAMAGE:
- wood cracks into cube shapes and crumbles away when dry
- leap-frogs through a house along non-wood materials, such as brick

TREATMENTS:
- cutting away infected wood and plaster to at least 60 cm beyond the decay
- cleaning and treating surrounding areas with fungicide
- installation of new, treated wood
- eradicating moisture and improving ventilation

Treat it right

Never be tempted to cut corners in the
treatment of dry rot. Cowboy operators will
happily take on the job then disappear into
the night, leaving you with no comeback
should this domestic cancer return – as it all
too often does after poor jobs. It is essential
to get a reputable company who will do a
fully guaranteed job, backed by an insurance
policy if necessary.

Wet Rot
. . . .

Not a destroyer on the same scale as dry rot,
wet rot is more commonly seen outdoors, for
example, in old wooden window frames or
other weather-battered woods.

Wet rot stops when the cause is treated. As
affected areas tend to be accessible and open
to the elements, it is usually fairly
straightforward to treat yourself.

Make sure you stay safe during any rot
treatment (see Danger! box, p.172).

WET ROT

CAUSES:
- repeatedly or naturally wet wood
- conditions need to be far wetter than those which let dry rot thrive

SIGNS:
- horizontal cracks along the wood with vertical cross-grain cracks forming cube shapes
- yellow-brown, dark brown or white strands may form on wood and wall

ASSOCIATED DAMAGE:
- timber rots by cracking and swelling; it remains open to moisture and further damage

TREATMENTS:
- removal of moisture source
- cutting away of rotted wood
- installation of new wood treated with fungicidal wood preservative; apply this to surrounding old wood, too
- for slightly damaged wood: paint on wood hardener, fill and paint as normal

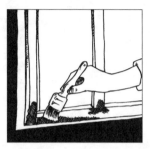

*Painting on wood hardener before filling and painting
(see Treatments, p.175)*

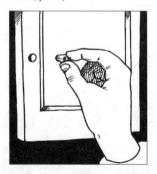

Preservative tablets help keep wood dry and rot-free

Preventing rot

Although you cannot totally eradicate the risk of a fungal or rot attack, there are steps you can take to guard against an outbreak.

Maintaining a rot-free property

- look after your home; an annual check-up will help alert you to damp problems (see Action! box, p.171)
- clean, paint and maintain door and window frames regularly
- protect wooden frames by inserting preservative tablets into drilled holes, before filling and painting
- ensure good ventilation under floors, above ceilings and in lofts
- eradicate plumbing faults quickly
- paint wood preservative on all exterior woods; check which type suits you as some harm plants

Damp: the causes

OUTDOOR SOURCES

- no damp-proof course
- faulty damp-proof course
- build-up of soil around a damp-proof course – it should be kept at least 15 cm below
- blocked ventilation outlets and airbricks
- damaged brickwork or mortar
- a leaky or faulty roof
- blocked, leaky and overflowing gutters
- leaky downpipes
- loose flashing on roofs or at chimneys

INDOOR SOURCES

- condensation

Damp

Damp is a potentially serious problem which can lead to rot if left untreated, and which can also pose a threat to your health.

Damp is always caused by something; the most common causes are listed in the box opposite. Once you have discovered the cause of dampness in a house, you can take steps to tackle it.

The two main types of dampness, dealt with in more detail on the following pages, are:

- rising damp
- penetrating damp

Condensation is a particular problem that can appear as either of these two types, and as an imbalance in a building's internal atmosphere and humidity. Ironically, insulation advances and the luxuries of modern living, such as en suite bathrooms, contribute to the problem.

RISING DAMP

SIGNS:
- problem is associated with solid floors and lower walls
- problem evident even in dry weather
- musty smells
- damp 'tide' marks on lower walls and at skirtings
- mould

ASSOCIATED DAMAGE:
- causes rot and mould if left untreated
- damages plaster
- ruins internal decor

TREATMENTS:
- repair or install damp-proof course (between the bricks) or damp-proof membrane (beneath a concrete floor)
- clear soil or other debris piled up around the lower walls (a damp-proof course should be 15 cm clear of the ground at all points)

PENETRATING DAMP

SIGNS:
- specific, well-defined damp patches: the site of the problem will indicate where to look for the cause
- problem evident in wet weather only

ASSOCIATED DAMAGE:
- damp patch on affected area
- causes rot and mould if left untreated

TREATMENTS:
- depends on identified cause: repair roof or flashing; re-point or replace cracked mortar or bricks; replace porous bricks; clear blocked gutters and replace broken ones; repair leaking or damaged downpipes or overflows; replace render or coping; repair old or damaged window and door seals; clear drip-groove under window sill; clear out bridged wall cavity

Condensation

Condensation is not a full-scale home emergency but it is a damp-associated problem and as such should be cleared up as soon as possible. But its cause can often be hard to pin-point or cure.

Its scientific explanation is that a house's interior moisture-laden air (from cooking, bathing, showering and even breathing) contacts with a substantially colder surface, such as a porcelain toilet or a window. The colder temperature turns the watery vapours back into liquid form again.

But condensation-causing imbalances in a house's atmosphere can come from any combination of problems with internal temperature, humidity, ventilation and insulation, and even from the season: condensation problems are usually worse in winter. Interfering with the wrong cause might just move the problem to another area, or even make it worse.

CONDENSATION

CAUSES:
- imbalance in a house's micro-climate, from one or more of several factors

SIGNS:
- general condensation
- mould
- blistering paint
- misted glass or water pooling at sill
- dampness around a particular problem area, e.g. walls, chimney breast

TREATMENTS:
- good ventilation in rooms
- efficient heating (not paraffin)
- balanced insulation: e.g. insulate walls if you have double-glazed windows
- particular treatments for specific problems: put silica gel between fogging-up secondary glazing; lag pipes if moisture gathers there; ventilate lofts where mould on roof timbers is evident; ventilate a sealed-up chimney if there is dampness at chimney breast

Flooding

Flooding brings a different type of invasion into your home, and one which is probably more instantly destructive than any. In spite of the risk, many people still prefer to live close to water; others have houses in low-lying areas liable to flooding when rain is heavy and rivers are swollen. In any case, there is little you can do about the location of your house in the short term, so if you face a flood threat, however remote, being prepared will help you stay safe and minimise the damage if or when an emergency comes.

Pre-flood planning

If your area has a history of flooding, prepare yourself for the worst. Gather the supplies listed opposite and store them away in a box, ready to get out if they are needed. Having these to hand will save valuable preparation time. Perishables, like tinned goods and batteries, should be changed every year.

Emergency Supplies Kit

- water containers, purifying tablets
- 3 days' tinned food for those staying
- can and bottle opener
- 2 pans
- non-breakable beakers, plates, cutlery
- bucket with supply of plastic bags (to use as disposable toilet liners)
- toilet paper
- disinfectant
- camp stove and fuel
- matches
- candles
- battery-operated radio
- torch and spare batteries
- first-aid kit (see Appendix II, p. 253)
- personal hygiene kit that can be used without water

The local council can advise what height flood waters usually rise to, so you can plan sandbag defences accordingly.

Flood Preparation Plan

1. Monitor radio and TV for updates
2. Turn off electricity and gas before floods hit
3. Fill baths, buckets and bottles with drinking water
4. Move upstairs with your supplies, changes of clothes and valuable
5. If sandbags are not issued, improvise with old bedding and binbags filled with earth. Block off exterior doors and lower windows if necessary
6. If possible evacuate young children and the elderly (only safe if floods are localised, not over a wide area)

During and after a flood

The best advice to follow when a flood hits your home is to stay put. The emergency services know where you are and can evacuate you if necessary. Your presence will also deter looters. Listen to your radio for reports and instructions, and use your own stored-up water supply: don't drink tap water in case the supply has been contaminated.

Remember, as you try to keep warm without electricity or gas, that several light layers of clothing will be more effective than one or two bulky ones.

DANGER!

Be very careful when cleaning out flood-wash debris from your property. The waters may have picked up glass, toxins, sewage and other hazards along the way and deposited them at your doorstep, so sweep or shovel out initially and wear stout boots and gloves as you clean.

After the flood is over, you will want to start clearing up straight away, but carry on listening to radio reports to find out when it is safe to switch power supplies back on, to drink tap water and to travel.

Freeze-Ups

Much of the advice given for Flooding from page 184 onwards, including the Emergency Supplies Kit, should also stand you in good stead for a mid-winter freeze-up.

Pre-freeze-up planning

Common sense dictates regular servicing of central heating and this is the time when it pays off. Keep your heating on in the night, and don't let the house cool down. Draught-exclusion around doors and windows cuts heat loss, so close the curtains, if necessary (but don't cut off all supplies of fresh air).

Loft insulation should not extend under your cold-water tank, and if you can spare a

heater during a freeze, leave it in the room
below the tank.

Of course, in a freeze-up, unlike a flood,
the last thing you will want to do is shut off
your power supplies, but heavy snowfalls
often bring down power cables, in any case.
If you have a solid-fuel fire, get in supplies
of fuel, fire-lighters and kindling at the start
of winter.

One thing you should not do is hoard food.
To state the obvious: snow does not last
forever and in all probability you won't
starve before it melts. Three or four days'
supply should be enough – most people have
far more than that in their homes in the
normal course of things.

During a freeze-up

As with flooding, you should monitor your
local broadcasts for advice and information.

If you only have a heat source in one
room, live there until things get back to

normal. It is important to maintain your body temperature, so take hot drinks regularly. Check on elderly neighbours and people living alone to make sure they are alright.

If you go out, dress appropriately in warm layers, with a hat and mitts. Canadians and other nationals who regularly cope with long, severe winters get through them by making the most of them. As long as you have power supplies to come back to, an energetic and nearby session of snow-clearing, sledging or even snowman-building will warm you up a lot better than hugging a radiator, and stop you going cabin-crazy.

Do not drive unless in an emergency and if you do, take a shovel, a blanket, a mobile phone, some chocolate and plenty of petrol. Stay in your car if you get stuck.

8 Stains & Cleaning

ACTION!

7 STEPS TO TREAT FABRIC STAINS

1 Be prepared – keep your own stain-removal kit handy

2 Act now – clean it before it sets

3 Be careful – if you are unsure of either stain or remedy, use cold water only

4 Clean it yourself – a washing machine's hot water may set some stains hard

5 Be aware – learn how to treat the three basic stain types

6 Do a test run – some delicate fabrics might react badly

7 Don't try too hard – more than two goes at removing a stain may damage a fabric

Successful Stain Removal
· ·

There can be few things more irritating than
having to throw out a favourite item of
clothing because of a stain that can't be
removed. And if this happens on a regular
basis then it can prove expensive to replace
them.

This chapter will, hopefully, allow you to
keep all your wardrobe clean and intact by
showing you how to treat all but the most
stubborn of stains.

The rules of stain removal

As the Action! box at the start of this chapter
shows (see p.191), there are some basic rules
to successful stain removal from fabrics,
carpets and soft furnishings. Most of the
seven steps are self-explanatory, but one or
two of them would benefit from a little more
detail.

Stain-removal kit

- a sponge to apply water or cleaner; cotton-wool balls can do this job on a small stain

- a white cloth or ripped-up white towel to pad behind stains as you clean

- white kitchen towel to blot up liquid messes

- a spoon or knife to scrape up solid spills

- a toothbrush to use on small stains or delicate fabrics

- cotton buds to treat small stains in difficult-to-get-to places

- a small, stiff-bristled clothes brush

- rubber gloves to protect your hands from any cleaners you use

Clean it immediately

It is very tempting just to drop stained clothes into the laundry basket and leave the washing machine to do all the cleaning for you, but you will already be fighting a losing battle if you let a stain dry in. If you are at home, abandon whatever else you are doing to deal with it on the spot. It's worth it in the long run.

To make sure you can react instantly when a staining accident happens, try to keep together, under the sink in an old plastic tub or microwave container, the 'tools' listed on p.193.

As well as a toolkit that will help you do the job properly, there are several store-cupboard ingredients that will let you treat most stains. These are listed on p.196 and followed by detailed instructions on their use.

The boxes on p.195 show the dangers of using chemicals, and sensible precautions to take when working with domestic cleaners.

DANGER!

Toxic chemicals poison in several ways:
- *absorption: liquids and powders can enter your body through your skin*
- *burns: chemicals that burn your skin can get into your bloodstream quickly*
- *ingestion: chemicals can get trapped in cracks in the hands or under nails*
- *inhalation: breathing in fumes or powder lets toxins into the lungs and blood*
- *sensitivity: prolonged exposure to a toxin heightens sensitivity to it and increases the likelihood of a future allergic reaction*

NEVER MIX ONE KIND OF CLEANER WITH ANOTHER – YOU COULD BE CREATING A DEADLY TOXIC COCKTAIL

✗ Don't work in food preparation areas
✔ Do wear rubber gloves and a face mask, if needed
✔ Do have good venitlation; work by a window
✔ Do wash hands and nails when you finish

Store-cupboard stain removers

- ammonia
- amyl acetate
- biological detergent
- borax (laundry)
- eucalyptus oil
- glycerine
- hydrogen peroxide
- lemon
- methylated spirit
- proprietary cleaners
- salt
- talcum powder
- washing soda
- washing-up liquid
- white spirit
- white vinegar

Ammonia General stain remover. Mix 1 teaspoon (tsp) to 0.5 litre (l) water. Test for colourfastness. Toxic.

Amyl acetate Breaks up nail polish, paint, grease and glue. Flammable; toxic.

Biological detergent Its enzymes make it effective on protein stains, from bodily fluids to milk, egg, etc. Soak in a solution with cold water; the exact concentration will be listed on each pack. Remove any metal trims before soaking. Do not use with delicate fabrics or special finishes. Irritant.

Borax (laundry) Halts acid action and is useful for acidic stains such as fruit juice and wine. Leaches colour out after 10–20 minutes, so it must be washed out. Mix 1 tablespoon (tbs) to 0.5 l warm water. Toxic.

Eucalyptus oil Useful on tar and grease stains. Irritant.

Glycerine Good for softening up dried-in marks. Dilute in equal parts with warm water and leave on the stain for at least half an hour. Glycerine solution should be washed off before you move on to the next step.

Hydrogen peroxide   With a milder action than bleach, this can be used on delicate fabrics but not those with a special finish. Dilute 20 volumes strength hydrogen peroxide 1:6 with water. Safest to use on white articles, as it may lift the colour out of coloured ones after only 20 minutes. Toxic.

Lemon   Acidity makes it a good, handy natural bleach. Useful for stains such as rust and fruit juice. Rub on the cut surface of a fresh lemon or use juice from a bottle. Lemon can leave its own stain on some fabrics.

Methylated spirit   Use neat to treat residual marks that are resistant to other stain-removal treatments. Do not use on acetates. Toxic.

Proprietary cleaners   You can buy dedicated cleaners in handy dispensers for virtually any stain you can think of. These are very good, but the main drawback is that unless you are organised enough to have bought a complete set, they will never be there when you actually need them. Convenience, versatility and relative cheapness is what makes this list of storecupboard cleaners so useful a substitute. It is always worth being prepared with the cleaners you will use most often, however: investing in a biological stick-cleaner and a pack of carpet wipes, for example, is never going to be a bad idea.

Salt Dissolve a handful in a bucket of cold water to loosen relatively light biological stains such as sweat and blood. Can also blot up stains.

Talcum powder Like salt, a good stain absorber. Use on water-soluble and fat stains. Irritant.

Washing soda Useful for fat stains on some fabrics. Irritant.

Washing-up liquid Use to mix up soapy water. A good multi-purpose cleaner.

White spirit Good for removing some paints, polishes and adhesives. Toxic.

White vinegar Can be used in place of a bleach solution, especially for non-washables.

Know the basic stain types

Although there are innumerable different types of stain, most of the main ones encountered in the home conform to three basic categories. Each of these calls for a quite different treatment:

- fat or grease stains

- protein stains

- water-soluble stains

In an emergency, where you don't have time to seek out specific stain advice, the following rules should be useful: residual fat stains will respond to hot soapy water; protein stains need cold-water rinsing and treatment with biological detergents; and water-soluble stains should be shifted by cold-water washing with a little soap if necessary.

More detailed stain treatments are listed from page 203 on.

Know the technique

Most types of stains on fabrics, soft
furnishings and carpets will respond to the
same basic technique. Following the rules
outlined below should help minimise any
further stain damage to fabrics.

Stain-removal technique

- work initially from the back of the
  fabric to push any residues off the
  fabric and on to your pad; working
  from the front may ingrain the problem

- always work from the outside in: this
  will avoid spreading the stain

- pad behind the area you are
  working on with a white cloth to
  soak up any water, cleaner and
  washed-out stain residues

- if you are using solvents, work by an
  open window to let the fumes dissipate

Special treatments

Some fabrics react badly to cleaners and even water may damage them. If you are unsure, test on an inconspicuous part of the fabric, like an inside seam, before treating the stain.

Those more likely to be temperamental include fabrics with a special finish, such as some curtain and upholstery fabrics, delicates, those labelled Dry Clean Only, some artificial fabrics and those with non-fast colours.

Proceed with care

The first piece of cleaning advice is to act quickly; the second is the maxim 'look before you leap'. If you are not sure how to treat a stain, don't just squirt washing-up liquid at it and hope for the best. Unless an item is marked Dry Clean Only, you will do little harm with plain cold water. At the very least this will dilute the stain, letting you blot off the worst of it, and keep it moist until you find its specific remedy.

A–Z of Stain Removal
••••••••••••••••••••••••

Adhesive

Ideally, you will have bought a solvent at the same time as you bought the adhesive, but in practice hardly anyone ever does. There are many different types of adhesive and almost as many stain-removing solutions.

The key to removing as much adhesive as you can is to do it while the stain is fresh. But you may still have to reconcile yourself to some sort of residual mark on the fabric. Begin by scraping off any surplus, pushing it out of the fabric from the back while you do so. Then wash the stain in water; with some adhesives, such as contact adhesives, this may wash out the stain.

Clear adhesive (e.g. UHU) Amyl acetone.
Contact adhesive (e.g. Evostick) Amyl acetone; methylated spirit.
Epoxy adhesive and resin Methylated spirit.
Latex adhesive (e.g. Copydex) Try the

manufacturer's solvent if you can get it, or white spirit. This adhesive can be removed from a hard surface by rolling it off with your fingers.

Superglue Immediate action is the key to removal from fabrics or skin; immerse in water, or soak with water-filled cloths for a long time, before the glue bonds – this should loosen it.

Beer

Sponge the stain with lukewarm water or, if this doesn't work, a solution of 1 part white vinegar to 5 parts water (not for acetates); wash as normal before it dries.

Treat carpet stains with a carpet shampoo.

For dried-in stains, dab gently with methylated spirit on a cloth.

Beetroot

Rinse the item under cold running water then soak it in a borax solution (see p.197). If the item is not washable, sponge it down with cold water to take out as much of the stain as possible before having it dry cleaned.

Blood

Fresh stains Soak items immediately in a cold-water salt solution (see p.199) before moving on to a soak in a biological detergent. Make sure the stain is completely removed before you wash the item in the washing machine, as hot water will set a protein stain such as blood.

Old stains A dried-in stain will need to be left overnight in cold water and biological detergent, or try dabbing it with an ammonia or hydrogen peroxide solution (see p.198).

Carpets Sponge repeatedly with cold water until the stain is gone then use carpet shampoo.

Mattresses Blood-stained mattresses should be tipped on their side then, with a towel held in place to stop water running down, wash the mattress with a salt-water solution. Once you are satisfied that the stain has gone completely, play a hairdryer on the watermark to help speed up the drying process.

Burn and scorch marks

Rub a washable fabric under cold running water then soak in a borax solution (see p. 197). If the fabric is not washable, sponge the stain gently with a borax solution.

For cigarette or other burns on carpets, either cut off the burnt tufts or rub the area with a fine sandpaper in a circular movement. Then treat as for non-washable fabrics.

Candle wax

Leave until the wax hardens, then scrape it off. Lay a paper towel under the stain, another over it and press with a warm iron; repeat continually, using clean pieces of towel to absorb the wax. Dab with methylated spirit to take out any discolouration.

Chewing gum

Pull off what you can then put the item in the freezer for a couple of hours. This should harden the gum enough for it to be broken off.

To treat a carpet, hold a freezer bag full of ice cubes over the chewing gum until it hardens, then pick it off.

Chocolate

Let the chocolate set hard then scrape off the excess. Dab glycerine onto the stain, leave it for 10 minutes then sponge it with water and a biological detergent.

On carpets, use a carpet shampoo.

Coffee

Coffee is a natural dye, so act quickly. Mop up the excess and rinse the item in warm water before soaking it in a warm-water biological detergent solution. If this doesn't work, apply a hydrogen peroxide solution (see p.198).

If the stain is on a carpet, sponge it with water before applying some carpet shampoo.

Crayons see Make-up

Creosote

Sponge eucalyptus oil onto washable items; non-washable ones will need to be dry-cleaned. Carpets and furnishings will also need professional treatment.

Curry

The turmeric in curry is a natural dye, and this is one of the hardest stains to shift.

Rinse in cool water, then apply glycerine to stop the stain setting. Leave this on for at least half an hour before washing in biological detergent. Apply a hydrogen peroxide solution to stubborn stains (see p. 198).

Furniture and carpet stains may be sponged down with a borax solution (see p.197), but professional cleaning may be the only answer.

Droppings see Excrement

Dye

Do not let a dye-stained fabric dry or get into hot water: either will set the colour forever.

Rinse the affected item in cold water then soak in a biological detergent solution. For delicates, apply a hydrogen peroxide solution (see p.198). Bleach or a colour-run remover will remove the stain but also the colour from the fabric, so you may only want to use this on whites. Alternatively, you could dye the garment's own colour back in afterwards.

Apply methylated spirits to isolated stains on fabrics or carpets. Treat splashes on the skin by rubbing on a cut lemon.

Egg

Try to treat egg stains before they harden. Scrape off any excess then sponge with salt water. As for most protein stains, soak in a biological detergent solution. If this doesn't work, dab on a borax solution (see p.197).

Non-washable items should be treated with cold salt water followed by a washing-up-liquid solution and a rinse with cold water.

On fabrics, soft furnishings and carpets such a tricky stain as this may call for a proprietary cleaner, such as Stain Devils.

Excrement and Droppings

Indoors On fabrics, furnishings and carpets, scrape up any excess. Soak clothes in biological detergent and treat residual stains with hydrogen peroxide solution (see p.198).

Carpets and furnishings can be sponged with ammonia solution (see p.197). Follow up with a carpet shampoo.

Outdoors Bird droppings may affect newly washed clothes. As before, take off the solids, then rinse out the stain in cold water. Hydrogen peroxide solution can lift off any residues; the item can be treated as normal.

If you get any bird droppings on your car,

wipe them off *immediately*. Droppings will indelibly stain a car's paintwork if they are not removed in two or three days, at most.

Fat

On any surface you should begin by blotting up as much as possible with paper kitchen towels before treating the stain.

Dab eucalyptus oil on fabric until the stain loosens. It can then either be washed out or, if dry-clean only, sponged with cool water.

On soft furnishings, talcum powder can be used as the blotter. Dust it all over the stain, leave for about 15 minutes then brush off. Repeat as necessary.

Carpets can be blotted with paper towels and a hot iron before using carpet shampoo.

Felt tips

On fabrics, carpets and furnishings, dab and blot on methylated spirit. Washable items should then be washed in soap and water.

Fruit juice

A natural dye. Blot off as much as possible onto paper towels then rinse the item under cold running water or rub a cut lemon onto the stain to counteract it. Methylated spirit or a borax solution (see p.197) are other options.

Dried-in stains should first be treated with glycerine to loosen them up, then the above methods applied.

Glue see Adhesive

Grass

White cotton can simply be left to soak in a bleach solution. For other fabrics, apply a proprietary stain remover or methylated spirit to the fabric before giving a cold-water rinse and washing as normal.

Ice cream

Scrape up the excess. Leave washable items to soak in biological detergent. Treat dried-in stains with a borax solution (see p.197).

Non-washable fabrics should be sponged with cool water then treated with a grease solvent before being dry cleaned. For carpets, follow this treatment but finish up with carpet shampoo in place of dry cleaning.

Ink (see also Felt tips)

There are several different types of ink, each responding to different treatments. Some of the following should work.

Soak or dab a washable item with milk, which draws out non-permanent inks (but then see the treatment for milk stains). Alternatives are to dab on either ammonia, a thick soapflake solution, methylated spirits, or lemon juice; each of these can be blotted off with a white cloth or paper towel.

Methylated spirits can also be used on non-washable fabrics and furnishings. For carpets, pour on salt to blot up the ink; vacuum it away before pouring on hot milk.

Finally, wash it all thoroughly with a hot soapy solution or carpet shampoo.

Jam and Preserves

Scrape up any residues. Soak washable items in biological detergent and if this doesn't work follow it with a borax solution (see p.197).

Non-washables and furnishings should be sponged with cold water then dabbed with either the borax solution or a washing-up liquid solution.

For carpets, carpet shampoo is best.

Ketchup

Rinse washable fabrics in fresh, cold water then soak in a hydrogen peroxide solution or dab on methylated spirits. On non-washables, try to blot off with water as much as you can before having the item dry cleaned.

Use carpet shampoo on carpets and soft furnishings, following up with a proprietary stain remover for persistent marks.

Make-up

Mascara A water-based eye-make-up remover, or just plain soap, or washing-up liquid, and water can be used on most types of mascara. The exception is waterproof, which should be dabbed with eucalyptus oil, then sponged with soap and water, as above.

For non-washable items, use a proprietary stain remover or, if the item is colourfast, dab on a special solution of ammonia: mix up 1 : 3 with water.

Lipstick The oils, waxes and dyes in lipstick make it one of the trickiest of everyday stains to deal with.

Treat with eucalyptus oil, blotting it on and reapplying if necessary. If this does not work, glycerine may also help shift it. On washable fabrics, blot on washing-up liquid then sponge it off with hot water.

Carpet shampoo or a proprietary dry-cleaning solvent will be needed on carpets or soft furnishings.

Foundation Blot off any excess then cover with talcum powder to soak up the oils. Brush this off and follow up by soaking in an ammonia solution. Wash as normal.

On dry-clean-only items, dab on a little methylated spirit after the talcum powder stage.

Nail Polish The obvious answer is a non-oily nail-polish remover dabbed on with cotton wool, but remover contains acetone which harms many acetate-based fabrics. Non-washable items should be cleaned professionally.

Milk

Another stain for which speed is of the essence, not for the mark it leaves, but for its trademark near-unshiftable baby-sick smell.

Sponge down carpets or furnishings with cool water and follow up with carpet or upholstery shampoo. If the smell still lingers on even after the stain has gone, you may need to have the item professionally cleaned.

For clothes, the usual remedy of a cold-water rinse and soak in biological detergent is the answer. Dry-clean-only items may need a proprietary stain remover.

Mould and mildew

These stains develop in areas of condensation or damp in the home – normally around window frames and in bathrooms. Mould and mildew can stain permanently, so if any surfaces in your house are prone to them, wipe them clean regularly with a bactericide specially designed for the job.

Washable items should be soaked in a hydrogen peroxide solution (see p.198), but keep a close eye on coloureds for any run. Alternatively, treat coloureds as nylon or lace fabrics: these should be rubbed with washing soap and left out in the sun for several hours. Waiting in vain for sunshine may be enough to persuade you to have the items dry cleaned.

Mud

Leave it to dry completely, then brush it off. Follow up with a normal wash if necessary.

Paint

It is vital to deal with paint stains as soon as they happen; once the paint dries you have virtually no chance of getting it out. Some paint manufacturers sell their own solvents; to be on the safe side, you may want to buy these at the outset if you plan to paint a lot.

Paints that are water-based, such as emulsion, can simply be washed out with soap and water. Oil-based paint, including gloss and lacquer, should be dabbed with white spirit or turpentine, with the process repeated as necessary.

Perfume

The alcohol in perfume can lift the dye out of some fabrics, so be careful how you use it.

If it spills, rinse the fabric immediately

then wash as usual; if the perfume has dried, apply glycerine, leave it for an hour then wash as normal.

For dry-clean-only items, apply glycerine then carefully sponge off with warm water.

Soft furnishings and carpets need to be sponged with warm water then cleaned with upholstery or carpet shampoo.

Plasticine

Scrape off any squashed-in plasticine before treating with a grease solvent. Some stains also respond well to a hot water and soap wash, but others will need to be dry cleaned.

Rust

Apply lemon juice, fresh or bottled, to the stain, then cover the juice mark with salt. Leave it aside for at least an hour, preferably in the sun, then check to see if the stain is gone – if not, squeeze on more lemon juice. Finally, brush the salt off and clean as normal.

This procedure should be used with care on delicates and some coloureds, as the lemon juice can lift the colour from some fabrics.

Scorch marks see Burn and scorch marks

Shoe Polish

Apply white spirit, repeating as often as is needed. When the stain has gone, wash out the white spirit in hot, soapy water.

Non-washable fabrics can also be treated with white spirit, but sponge it off gently with water. The treatment also works for carpets and furnishings.

Sick

Working as always from the outside in, scrape up all the solids before starting to treat the stain.

For stains on carpets, if you do not have carpet shampoo to hand sponge the area with a borax solution (see p.197) followed by lukewarm water containing some disinfectant. Follow up with a carpet shampoo. Repeated treatments may be needed to get rid of the smell.

Rinse washable items under cold running water, then soak in a biological detergent and disinfectant solution; wash as normal.

Dry-clean-only fabrics should be sponged with lukewarm water containing some ammonia, then cleaned as normal.

Sweat

Perspiration marks, especially at the underarms, can ruin otherwise perfectly good clothes.

Dissolve a handful of salt in a bucket of cold water as a soak to loosen relatively light sweat stains. If the dye has already run, try sponging them with a white vinegar solution (1 tablespoon vinegar to a 0.3 litre of warm water); alternatively, apply an ammonia solution (see p.197). Then soak in a biological

detergent, or have non-washable fabrics
professionally dry-cleaned.

Tar

These stains may be found more often on
carpets than clothes, as people drag tar in on
their shoes.

Eucalyptus oil is the safest and most
effective remedy for tar stains. Dab it on,
blotting it off from the stain side. When the
stain is removed, sponge the remaining oil
away with soap and water.

Tea

As with almost any stain, these are best dealt
with while they are fresh; dried-in tea stains
are quite tricky to shift.

For fresh stains, soak the item in a borax
solution (see p.197) followed by a biological
detergent soak and wash as normal.

Older stains should be softened up with
glycerine for a few hours, then sponged with

a borax solution. If this still doesn't work, dab on methylated spirit. Lemon juice also removes tea stains, at some risk to the colours, but you may find you need to bleach the article to get stains out completely.

Carpet, furnishings and dry-clean-only items should be sponged with borax then treated with a proprietary stain remover.

Urine

Quick action is needed to avoid lingering smells and stains.

Rinse out washable items in cold water, follow with a biological detergent soak then wash as normal.

Non-washable items should simply be sponged down, first with cold water then with a white-vinegar solution (1 teaspoon of distilled white vinegar to 0.5 litre of water). Wash out by sponging again with cold water.

Old urine stains may need soaking in a hydrogen peroxide solution (see p.198);

alternatively, try a proprietary stain remover.

Urine-stained mattresses should be treated as outlined at *Blood*.

Wine

Red If the wine spills on a tablecloth, soak up any excess with white paper towels, then cover the stain with salt to blot it up.

On carpets, pour white wine over, making sure the original stain is fully covered. Sponge any remainder with warm water, then pat dry. If you have no white wine handy, use mineral water or even tap water – although neither is quite so effective as white wine.

The carpet treatment can also be used on clothes; alternatively, a rinse in warm water may work on fresh stains. Dry-clean-only items can be blotted with talcum powder before being professionally cleaned.

White White wine can be rinsed or dry-cleaned out of table linen, carpets and fabrics with relative ease.

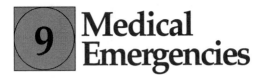

9 Medical Emergencies

First Aid

First Aid is a huge subject and much of it is beyond the scope of this volume. Ideally, every household should have at least one good First Aid manual which can be referred to when needed but if yours doesn't, you will at least find here brief summaries of the key actions you need to take to cope successfully with a range of **major** medical emergencies that can confront you in the home.

Attitude

As with all emergencies, the ability to keep calm in the face of a difficult and stressful situation, particularly one in which people may be seriously injured, is a great asset. Of course, this is easy to say but very difficult to do when under pressure. However, knowing what to do in a crisis can give you confidence and the ability to act calmly and efficiently. So, even if you don't do so for any other chapter in this book, read and rehearse the techniques listed in this one **before** you need to use them for real. Someone's life may depend on it.

✘ Don't put yourself in unnecessary danger. You will be little use to anyone if you also become injured

✘ Don't panic. Approach the situation calmly but don't waste time – seconds can count

✘ Don't attempt too much. Use what knowledge you have – and common sense – to do the best you can in the circumstances. Preventing the casualty's condition from worsening should be your goal

✘ Don't show any alarm or fears you may have to the casualty

✔ Do reassure the injured that you can handle
the situation or that medical staff will be
able to. At all times, try to relax the casualty

✔ Do enlist the help of others if you can (but
don't waste time looking for assistance)

Emergency Priorities

Regardless of the specific causes or effects of
a medical emergency, your immediate
concerns for anyone who is injured should be:

- that their airway is clear

- that they can breathe

- that they have a pulse

- that there is no bleeding from arteries

- that they are immobilised if you suspect
  a neck injury

By following the First Aid ABC, you will
fulfill the essentials required to ensure these
primary needs are met.

A is for an open Airway

Does the casualty respond when you speak to them? Are they moving? If not, **shout for help.** Then, check that the casualty is breathing by

- looking to see if their chest moves
- listening for breath sounds
- feeling for breath on your cheek

If the casualty is breathing

If the casualty is unconscious but breathing, put them in the recovery position (see p.236) then summon professional help.

If the casualty is not breathing

Tilt their head back and check again to see if the person is breathing; if not, lay them on their back and check for obvious reasons, e.g. vomit, false teeth or another obstruction in the mouth; unconsciousness also can cause the tongue to fall back over the airway. Turn the head to one side and clear away any loose objects or debris you find but be careful not to push anything further into the throat. If you still can't detect any signs of breathing:

- gently lift under the casualty's neck while pressing down on the forehead to tilt the head back

- while maintaining gentle pressure on the forehead, lift the chin upwards (the jaw will lift the tongue clear of the airway)

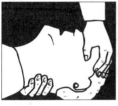 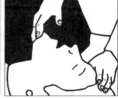

B is for adequate Breathing

If the casualty does not now begin breathing of their own accord, you must act fast to re-establish their natural breathing rhythm. **This takes priority over any other problem.**

ACTION!

MOUTH-TO-MOUTH RESUSCITATION

1 Keep the casualty's head tilted back and the chin up

2 Pinch the nostrils together to seal them (below left)

3 Seal the casualty's open mouth with yours and breathe deeply 4 times into it

4 Check that the chest wall rises with each breath (below right). If it doesn't, check again that the airway is clear and that you've remembered to pinch the nostrils (easily forgotten)

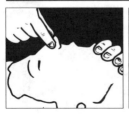
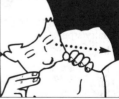

Resuscitating children If you have to give mouth-to-mouth to children, the technique is basically the same as that for adults except that it should be faster and gentler.

Under 2s: Open the airway as for adults but don't tilt the head too far back. Seal the mouth and nose with your mouth and puff in gently at the rate of 1 breath every 2 seconds.

Over 2s: Seal the mouth or nose or both depending on the child's size and puff air in as for the under-2s. After the first couple of inflations, check for a heart beat; you should feel a pulse on the inside of an upper arm or directly over the heart.

C is for proper Circulation

Having given the 4 breaths, check the casualty's pulse to see if their heart is beating and blood is circulating. The pulse can be felt by pressing gently using the tips of two fingers on either of the following three positions:

- the front of the wrist, about 1–2 cm back from the wrist joint on the thumb side

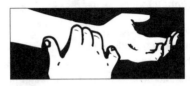

- the side of the neck, in the depression alongside the voicebox

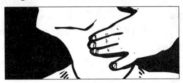

- directly over the heart

If the heart is beating, then there should be other signs besides the pulse, such as the casualty's colour returning: pink/red is good while blue or white is bad. If the heart is beating, continue mouth-to-mouth until the casualty begins to breathe for themselves or until professional help arrives. Continue checking the pulse every minute or so.

Cardiopulmonary resuscitation (CPR)

If you cannot find a pulse **and** the casualty isn't breathing then CPR will be necessary. This is a double-action procedure comprising mouth-to-mouth ventilations to restore breathing used in conjunction with chest compressions to re-start the heart and restore the pulse.

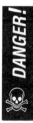

DANGER!

> NEVER perform chest compressions if the heart is still beating, however faintly, as it can stop the heart. CPR is a precise technique that requires practice and experience to be most effective.

Mouth-to-mouth resuscitation of the casualty should be performed as described on p.230 and if there is still no pulse, compress the casualty's chest in the way described overleaf.

CHEST COMPRESSION

1 Kneeling at one side of the casualty's chest, place your hands, one covering the other, on his or her breastbone

2 With your arms as straight as possible, press down quickly 15 times at half-second intervals. For an adult, apply only sufficient pressure to compress the chest wall by 4–5 cm

3 Follow this with another 2 mouth-to-mouth ventilations

4 Continue this combination. After every 4th combination, check for movement and breathing. If signs of life recur, continue mouth-to-mouth alone until breathing restarts

This technique is illustrated opposite.

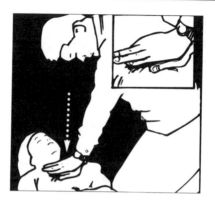

CPR with 2 people

If there are two people dealing with the casualty, one should go for help before helping with the CPR. One person should take charge of each function and you should aim for a ratio of 5 compressions to 1 ventilation. Time your efforts: be sure not to try to inflate the chest while it is being compressed by the other person.

CPR on children

If the casualty is a child, the chest should
only be compressed by about 2 cm and the
ratio should be 15 compressions to 2
ventilations. For an infant, use two fingers
pressing on the breastbone rather than the flat
of the whole hand as for adults; the ratio is as
for older children.

The Recovery Position

If the casualty is unconscious but is breathing
adequately and has a pulse, place them in the
recovery (or coma) position to ensure that
they will not choke.

The recovery position is illustrated
opposite. Be sure to position the limbs
correctly as shown to help maintain the body
in this posture. Also ensure that the head is
tilted back to ensure that the casualty's
airway remains open.

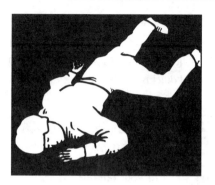

Specific Emergencies

The following list of specific medical conditions and how to treat them is not intended to cover every possible 'emergency' scenario that can confront you at home. However, the more common serious conditions are featured and the treatment descriptions given are intended to stabilise the casualty's state while professional help is sought.

Severe Bleeding

External bleeding

Heavy bleeding from a wound has to be stopped quickly to prevent shock (see p.251).

ACTION!

DIRECT PRESSURE

1 With casualty at rest, press down firmly on the wound with any clean, absorbent material or your bare hands. Hold the edges of the wound together if necessary. Maintain pressure for up to 15 min. to allow clotting

2 If a limb is bleeding, if possible raise it above the level of the heart (lie the casualty down)

3 If anything is embedded in the wound, DO NOT REMOVE IT – apply pressure around it

4 If blood seeps through a dressing, add another on top of the first

Pressure points

Where there is bleeding from an artery (where the blood is bright red and spurts in time to the heart beat) then indirect pressure to the artery feeding the injured limb can be effective. The main two arterial pressure points are

- on the middle of the inner side of the upper arm

- midway between the groin and the top of the thigh

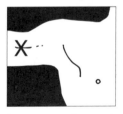
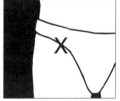

Pressure on these points must be released momentarily every minute and whenever bleeding stops without pressure.

ACTION!

INDIRECT PRESSURE FOR AN ARM WOUND

1 If possible raise the limb above the level of the head

2 Press firmly (inwards and upwards) on the arm pressure point, between the muscles, to trap the artery against the bone

3 Watch the rate of blood loss and adjust your pressure until it stops

INDIRECT PRESSURE FOR A LEG WOUND

1 With the casualty lying flat, raise the knee of the wounded limb and press on the leg pressure point, in the centre of the skin crease

2 Watch the rate of blood loss and adjust your pressure until it stops

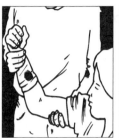
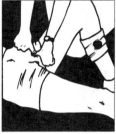

DANGER!

Don't apply pressure at a pressure point for more than 15 minutes or the loss of blood to the entire limb may lead to permanent damage or even amputatation

Burns and scalds

All but minor burns are potentially serious.
Deep burns and scalds can be identified by

- dark red, blistered or charred skin

- a loss of sensation in the burn area

ACTION!

CLOTHING ON FIRE

1 Lie the person down

2 Smother the flames with a coat, blanket or other heavy material

3 Once the flames are out, rapidly cool the casualty by pouring buckets or jugs of cold water over the affected areas for at least 10 minutes

4 Check the airway is clear (p.228) and phone the emergency services

5 Cover the burns with clean dressings if you have them (clean, non-fluffy, pillowcases can be used)

6 Give the casualty regular sips of cold water (only if they are conscious)

7 If the burned area is extensive, treat the casualty for shock (see Action! box, p.242)

ACTION!

BURNS AND SCALDS

1 Remove any clothes covering the burned area, except for fragments that are seared to the skin

2 Hold the burned area under running water for at least 10 mins

3 DO NOT apply butter or any lotions to the burn

4 DO NOT burst blisters. These should be covered with sterile dressings

CHEMICAL BURNS

1 Remove any chemicals to safety

2 Thoroughly wash the affected area under running water; brush off dry chemicals first

3 Remove contaminated clothing

4 Cover the burn with a clean dressing if it is inflamed

5 Get the casualty to hospital

CHEMICAL BURNS TO THE EYE

1 Thoroughly wash the affected eye under running water for as long as possible, letting the water run into the eye but not onto an unaffected eye. If both eyes are affected, alternate their washing for 10 sec. each

2 Ensure that the eyelids are kept apart, holding them yourself if necessary

3 Cover the affected eye with a sterile or clean dressing

4 Get the casualty to hospital

Burns to the mouth

If the casualty's mouth or throat has been burned or scalded and they are conscious, give them sips of cold water, ice cream or ice-cubes to suck and get them to a hospital.

Choking

Where a person is conscious and choking, first check inside their mouth for any obvious obstruction and remove it, if possible, taking care not to push it further into the airway. If this fails, slap the person sharply four times between the shoulder blades with the heel of your hand. Bending the person over while you do this helps; if the casualty is a child, bend them over your lap or, if an infant, rest them face down on your forearm with their head and chest supported by your hand.

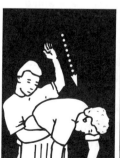
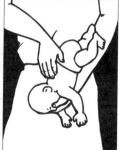

Abdominal thrusts

If the blockage persists, then try abdominal thrusts to remove it.

CHOKING: IF UPRIGHT AND CONSCIOUS

1 Stand behind the person with your arms around their waist

2 Clench one fist and position it with the thumb side against their abdomen, slightly above the navel. Place your other hand over the fist

3 Give 3 or 4 strong pulls, upwards and towards you, into their abdomen using your hands to create the thrust

If the casualty is an infant: Conscious or not, lay the baby down on her back and and press gently but firmly with the tips of two fingers just above her navel. Repeat up to 4 times.

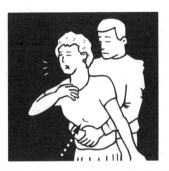

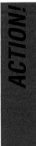

CHOKING: IF UNCONSCIOUS

1 Lie the casualty on his back and kneel astride him

2 Place the heel of one hand below the breastbone and cover it with your other hand

3 Give 4 strong thrusts inwards and upwards (see figure over)

4 Check and clear out the mouth after each thrust

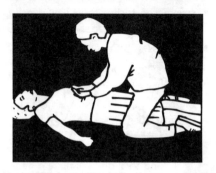

Electrocution

For details on how to cope with casualties who have been electrocuted, see p.63.

Gassing

For details on how to cope with casualties who have been overcome by fumes, see p.60.

Heart Attack

The typical warning signs of this condition are:

- ◉ severe, constricting chest pain which may spread to the throat, shoulders and arms
- ◉ shortness of breath and a weak or irregular pulse
- ◉ shock-like symptoms (see p.251)
- ◉ the casualty may collapse and fall into unconsciousness

ACTION!

SUSPECTED HEART ATTACK

1 Ring 999 and tell them a heart attack is suspected

2 If conscious, lie the casualty down with their knees slightly raised and loosen his clothing at the neck and chest

3 Check the breathing and pulse

4 If he becomes unconscious, place him in the recovery position (p.236)

5 If his breathing stops, use mouth-to-mouth (p.230). If the heart stops, start chest compression (p.234)

Poisoning

ACTION!

1 Ring 999 immediately

2 Gather as much information as possible about the poison and when it was taken (collect the bottle, container or plant)

3 If the casualty's mouth is burned, and they are conscious, make them drink water or milk slowly

4 Check pulse and breathing

5 If his breathing stops, use mouth-to-mouth (p.230). If the heart stops, start chest compression (p.234)

DANGER!

Don't make the casualty deliberately vomit. If using mouth-to-mouth, make sure the casualty's mouth is thoroughly cleaned of poison.

Shock

Typical warning signs of this condition are:

- pallid skin that feels moist and cold
- fast, shallow breathing and a rapid but weak pulse
- dizziness, blurred vision, thirst and nausea
- the casualty may become unconscious

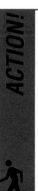

ACTION!

1 Lie the casualty down and treat any obvious injury causing the shock

2 Keep the head low, and raise and support the legs with a blanket

3 Reassure him and keep him inactive

4 Cover the casualty to keep him warm

5 Check pulse and breathing at regular intervals. If his breathing stops, use mouth-to-mouth (p.230). If the heart stops, start chest compression (p.234)

Appendix I: The Essential Home Tool Kit

For most of the domestic repair jobs you will need to do in an emergency, a basic tool kit of around a dozen items is all you need. These can easily be kept together in a small box:

- 1 small and 1 medium single-slot screwdriver
- 1 small and 1 medium Phillips or cross-headed screwdriver
- 1 small saw
- 1 small hacksaw with a spare blade
- Stanley knife or other craft knife
- pliers
- adjustable spanner, or a set of spanners
- claw hammer
- assorted screws and nails
- WD 40 or other lubricating oil

Appendix II: The Essential First Aid Kit

You can buy a ready-made first aid kit from a chemist's or make up your own. In either case, the kit should include at least:

- 2 triangular bandages (for slings and wounds)
- 2 crepe or open-weave bandages (to bind dressings and support joints)
- 2 large and 2 small sterile dressings
- 1 sterile eye dressing
- 4 gauze pads (as extra padding over a dressing)
- 1 packet of sterile cotton wool swabs
- assorted adhesive dressings or plasters
- 1 roll elastoplast
- 6 safety pins
- scissors and tweezers
- 1 packet of paracetamol tablets

Appendix III: Safe Asbestos Removal

Intact asbestos in your home is not an immediate hazard, but you could create one if you try to break or remove it yourself. Any breaks make asbestos friable (crumbly and flaky) – avoid this at all costs. Always get asbestos disposal advice from your local environmental health department.

This deadly substance is still commonly present in the fabric of older properties and in household goods; look out for it in:

- older appliances including toasters, hair dryers, irons (and ironing-board rests), tumble dryers, oven walls and seals, storage heaters, simmering pads

- oven gloves and fire blankets

- older textured ceiling and wall coverings

- wall cladding and insulation

- ceiling tiles and garage and outbuilding roofs

DANGER!

ASBESTOS FACTS

- Asbestos fibres are miniscule, sharp and long-lasting. They embed themselves in human tissue
- Asbestos fibres float in the air for up to 20 hours after being disturbed
- There is no safe level of exposure to asbestos fibres and dust
- One episode of exposure is all that is needed to trigger mesothelioma, the deadly lung-lining cancer associated with asbestos. Asbestosis and lung cancer can also result. Smokers, with their reduced lung capacity, are especially at risk

✗ Don't ever scrub, sand, saw or drill asbestos
✗ Don't ever remove or dispose of it yourself
✔ Do check regularly any asbestos in your home for signs of wear and tear

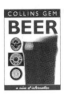 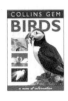

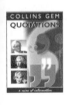   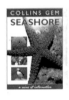